# Otolaryngology for the Pediatrician

## Editor

### Rahul K. Shah

*Associate Professor of Otolaryngology and Pediatrics*

## Co-Editors

### Diego A. Preciado

*Associate Professor of Otolaryngology and Pediatrics*

## &

### George H. Zalzal

*Professor of Otolaryngology and Pediatrics*
*Children's National Medical Center*
*George Washington University*
*111 Michigan Avenue, NW*
*Washington, D.C. 20010*

# CONTENTS

# FOREWORD

Otolaryngology is at home in the practice of Pediatrics, with common disorders in uncommon patients and uncommon disorders in common patients filling many of the moments in both primary and specialty care pediatrics. The broad spectrum of Otolaryngology disorders are seen at every developmental stage, from before birth – with congenital causes of upper airway obstruction, to choanal atresia presenting at birth to the ear infections of early childhood and neck masses and thyroid disorders seen in teens. These problems are best approached through coordinated care and interdisciplinary thinking.

The eminent authors of this volume seek to elucidate and amplify these themes through their chapters in this eBook. The electronic format should facilitate rapid access and referencing, and promote better outcomes for children seen with otolaryngology disorders, and in maintaining the much travelled bridge between the worlds of otolaryngology and pediatrics.

*Udayan K. Shah MD, FAAP, FACS*
Director, Fellow and Resident Education
Nemours/Alfred I duPont Hospital for Children
Wilmington, Delaware
Associate Professor of Otolaryngology-Head & Neck Surgery and Pediatrics
Thos. Jefferson University
Philadelphia, PA

# PREFACE

It is commonly known that many diseases and conditions of concern to the pediatric patient manifest in the region of the head, neck, ear, nose, and throat. As such, Otolaryngologists frequently work in partnership with their Pediatrics colleagues in the diagnosis and management of such conditions. Indeed, the sub-specialty of Pediatric Otolaryngology is relatively young – flourishing in the last three to four decades. Advances in Pediatric Otolaryngology have come from an international collaboration focused on tackling complex diagnostic and surgical issues in less than ideal conditions (small anatomy, underlying genetic malformations, limitations of instrumentation, *etc.*).

This eBook is written by eminent Pediatric Otolaryngologists chosen by the Editors for their specific research and clinical expertise in the conditions that they discuss. Each chapter provides a succinct overview of the clinical problem and its pertinence for the Pediatrician in managing such conditions. As expected, these are intended to be cursory discussions and of high clinical relevance for our colleagues.

We sincerely appreciate the efforts of our authors and the publisher in helping this vision of an eBook dedicated to specific pediatric Otolaryngology conditions come to fruition. We are eager to share this with our health professional colleagues across the world and sincerely hope you find the content of pertinence and interest to the care you all provide.

*Rahul K. Shah*
Associate Professor of Otolaryngology and Pediatrics

*Diego A. Preciado*
Associate Professor of Otolaryngology and Pediatrics

*George H. Zalzal*
Professor of Otolaryngology and Pediatrics
Children's National Medical Center
George Washington University
111 Michigan Avenue, NW
Washington, D.C. 20010

# List of Contributors

**Cristina Baldassari**

Children's Hospital of Kings Daughters, 601 Children's Lane, Norfolk, VA 23507, USA

**Nancy M. Bauman**

Children's National Medical Center, 111 Michigan Avenue, NW, Washington, D.C. 20010, USA

**Scott E. Brietzke**

Department of Otolaryngology, Walter Reed National Military Medical Center, Bethesda, MD, USA

**Robert H. Chun**

Department of Otolaryngology and Communication Sciences, Children's Hospital of Wisconsin, 9000 W Wisconsin Ave, Milwaukee, Wisconsin 53226, USA

**Craig Derkay**

Children's Hospital of the King's Daughters, Eastern Virginia Medical School, Norfolk, Virginia, USA

**Charles Elmaraghy**

Assistant Clinical Professor, Nationalwide Children's Hospital, Department of Otolaryngology, Ohio State University Medical Center, 700 Children's Drive, Columbus, OH 43205, USA

**Jan Groblewski**

Hasbro Children's Hospital, Providence, RI 02903, USA

**Diego A. Preciado**

Children's National Medical Center, 111 Michigan Avenue, NW, Washington, D.C. 20010, USA

**Brian Reilly**

Children's National Medical Center, 111 Michigan Avenue, NW, Washington, D.C. 20010, USA

**Rahul K. Shah**

Children's National Medical Center, 111 Michigan Avenue, NW, Washington, D.C. 20010, USA

**Sven-Orlik Streubel**

Assistant Professor, The Children's Hospital Otolaryngology, 13123 E. 16th Avenue, B455, Aurora, CO 80045, USA

**George H. Zalzal**

Children's National Medical Center, 111 Michigan Avenue, NW, Washington, D.C. 20010, USA

# Otolaryngology for the Pediatrician

Send Orders of Reprints at reprints@benthamscience.net

*Otolaryngology for the Pediatrician*, 2013, 3-24       **3**

# CHAPTER 1

## Clincal Anatomy for the Pediatrician

### Robert Chun[*] and Opeyemi Daramola

*Children's Hospital of Wisconsin, Department of Otolaryngology/ Medical College of Wisconsin, Children's Hospital Clinics Building, 9000 West Wisconsin Avenue, Suite 540, P.O BOX 1997, Milwaukee, Wisconsin 53226, USA*

**Abstract:** The anatomy of the head and neck is rich in depth and detail. This chapter explores the fundamentals of otolaryngologic anatomy and discusses common pathologies associated with each section. The chapter is separated in sections discussing the ears, nasal cavity, oral cavity and oropharynx, the neck and the larynx.

**Keywords:** External Ear, Middle Ear, Inner Ear, Oropharynx, Oral Cavity, Neck, Larynx, Nasal cavity, Sinus, Anterior triangle, Posterior Triangle.

## EAR

Diseases of the ear are common reasons for visits to the pediatrician's office. To understand the pathophysiology of otologic disease, an understanding of ear anatomy is essential. The ear has three parts: the external ear, middle ear and inner ear. This section provides a description of the different parts of the ear and how these parts contribute to hearing and balance in the growing child or adolescent.

## EXTERNAL EAR

The external ear consists of the auricle and external auditory canal (EAC). The auricle may also be referred to as the pinna. The pinna has cartilaginous and

─────────────────────────────────────────────
*\*Address correspondence to Robert Chun:* Children's Hospital of Wisconsin, Department of Otolaryngology/ Medical College of Wisconsin, Children's Hospital Clinics Building, 9000 West Wisconsin Avenue, Suite 540, P.O BOX 1997, Milwaukee, Wisconsin 53226, USA; Tel: 414-266-8383; Fax: 414-266-2693; E-mail: rchun@mcw.edu

noncartiliaginous portions. The noncartilaginous portion, located in the inferior portion of the pinna, is named the lobule. The basic but important purpose of the pinna is to direct sound to the middle and inner ear. The pinna amplifies sound to the middle ear by 6-10 decibels. It also serves an aesthetic purpose as parents may seek consultation for noted auricular asymmetry or congenital malformation of the pinna. The EAC is also subdivided into an "outer" third cartilaginous section and an inner two third bony section which adjoins the ear drum/tympanic membrane.

Notable malformation and diseases of the external ear that a pediatrician may encounter include microtia, preauricular tag or pit, cerumen impaction/ear wax, perichondritis, trauma and otitis externa.

Microtia refers to underdevelopment or absence (anotia) of the pinna. This is unilateral 80% of the time and occurs in 1 out of 6000 births. When the EAC is absent or malformed as well, this is known as canal atresia. When EAC atresia is recognized, the child should be referred for a full hearing evaluation and amplification. While the child will have a degree of conductive hearing loss, formal testing of hearing is recommended to screen for associated sensorineural hearing loss. The child can then be fitted with the necessary hearing amplification. Careful physical examination must be performed at all visits to screen for associated syndromes. However, as mentioned above, co management with a pediatric otolaryngologist who specializes in this malformation is ideal.

Preauricular tags or pits are developmental anomalies of the brachial arches and are often located anterior to the auricle. These are often normal and require no intervention. However, preauricular pits may occasionally become infected and result into an abscess requiring surgical drainage and antibiotic therapy. They may also be associated findings with some forms of hearing loss and renal anomalies. Thus, children with noted tags and/or pits, with hearing loss, should be referred to an Otolaryngologist for further care and continued surveillance. Furthermore, pits may actually be sinus tracts that may be connected to the middle ear. These anomalies are regarded as first branchial cleft anomalies. Surgical treatment is often curative for these lesions.

Perichondritis is inflammation or cellulitis of the cartilaginous portion of the auricle. The auricle becomes swollen, erythematous and exquisitely tender to palpation. There is no fluctuance and the lobule is unaffected. Therapy includes use of antibiotics, warm or cold compresses, and anti-inflammatory medications.

Auricular hematoma is another common pathology that a pediatrician may be presented. It represents an accumulation of clot between the subperichondrial space. Thus, the cartilage is separated from its blood supply. History is characterized by blunt force or sports such as wrestling. The hematoma should be drained widely using a scalpel within 48-72 hours and a bolster must be placed for 1-2 weeks to prevent reorganization of hematoma. Untreated auricular hematoma and perichondritis can lead to cartilaginous deformities and a "cauliflower" ear.

Cerumen or earwax impaction can have significant impact on the quality of life of children and adults alike. Cerumen is expected to migrate laterally and exit the canal without instrumentation. However, if there is overproduction of cerumen or stenotic ear canals to the extent that it causes hearing loss, pain, or precludes proper assessment of hearing, then it should be removed. This may be performed in the office using suction, irrigation with warm water. A word of caution - vigorous irrigation can potentially lead to tympanic membrane perforation or damage to the middle ear structures. Challenging cases may be started on otic drops for dissolution or softening of the cerumen. Alternatively, children suspected of external ear or middle ear disease whom must have an objective assessment of their hearing completed should be referred to an Otolaryngologist for cerumen removal under the microscope.

Another situation that may require otomicroscopy is foreign body in the ear. These are actually common in the emergency setting although they do not always require emergent intervention. Batteries, however, must be removed immediately due to rapid outset of skin necrosis. The foreign bodies include stones, beads, toys, vegetable, cotton, pencils, and insects. Objects may be retrieved in the office using an operating otoscope and instruments such as alligator forceps, suction and wire loupes. Irrigation may also be used for the nonperforated ear although this may cause significant distress. Vegetative matter should not have drops or irrigation due to subsequent swelling. Insects may be killed with mineral oil, lidocaine solution (2%) and suctioned out or removed manually in a piecemeal fashion. A referral should be placed to an ear specialist for consultation if the canal has been traumatized by attempts at removal or a fast retrieval (batteries) is indicated.

Acute otitis externa can be a challenging diagnosis for the primary care provider because of the need to differentiate this disease from otitis media. Otitis externa refers to infection of the external auditory canal skin. It is may be seen when there are conditions that promote water (swimmer's ear) and debris. Ototopical drops with steroids usually will treat the disease. Trauma to the external auditory canal (EAC) skin also promotes bacterial invasion. Malignant otitis externa is a spread of the otitis externa to the surrounding bone and cartilage. Children who are diabetic and immuno-compromised are at a higher risk. Clinical symptoms include pain, edema of the EAC canal that may preclude otoscopic visualization of the ear drum. In fact, examination on initial presentation may be very difficult secondary to pain. Most common pathogens include *Pseudomonas aeroginosa, Staphyloccocus aureus* and Streptococcus species.

Patients present with one or more of the following: history of 1-3 days of pain, pruritus, purulent discharge, hearing loss, fullness or pressure and history of recent exposure to water during recreational or sporting activities. On exam, gentle traction or pulling of the auricle elicits pain. There is edema of the EAC canal and often debris that requires some gentle aural toilet with soft wire loops or careful suction with Frazier tip suction. A good attempt should be made to visualize the tympanic membrane. Exam may be limited but pnuemo-otoscopy can help identify concomitant otitis media as the ear drum often appears normal and moves readily in isolated otitis externa.

Treatment for otitis externa consists of medical treatment and ear canal debridment. A wick may be necessary to deliver drugs to the entire EAC if there is significant edema of the EAC. If bleeding, granulation tissue, failure to improve on ototopical drops, disease with an immuno-compromised patient, or suspected advancement of disease with bony erosion (malignant otitis media), then the referral for immediate otolaryngology assessment should be placed.

The tympanic membrane (TM) represents the medial extent of the external ear. It measures about 9-10mm in diameter and has a concave appearance on otoscopy. The tissue is thin and skin-like with less tolerance for insults relative to the EAC skin itself. It serves to help transmit and amplify sound. It also protects the contents of the middle ear. The TM may become inflamed (myringitis) secondary to trauma, foreign body, infection or eczema. The myringitis may also be concurrent with an episode of acute otitis media. The underlying cause of inflammation should be addressed. Otic drops should be initiated as well.

Perforation of the tympanic membrane (TM) due to trauma usually heals spontaneously. However, dizziness or vertiginous symptoms may indicate injury to the inner ear structures and potential perilymphatic leak. While most minor perforations heal, persistent tympanic membrane perforations may cause mild conductive hearing loss and may require surgical management.

## MIDDLE EAR

The middle ear consists of the space between the TM and cochlea, the three bones of the middle ear (ossicles), and muscles that contribute to transmission of sound from the outer ear to the cochlea (inner ear). There is a connection between the middle ear and the nasal cavity: this is known as the Eustachian tube (ET). The ET is important for maintenance of pressure between the middle ear and the outside atmosphere. Dysfunction of this tube may result in aural fullness, and predisposition to otitis media. As the child grows the ET elongates and increases in angle improving its function. While the ET still grows, children with short and flat ET have an anatomical predisposition for ear infections.

Ossicles transmit sound pressure from the tympanic membrane to the inner ear. They consist of the malleus, incus and stapes. The malleus is attached to the TM and the stapes is connected to the cochlea. These ossicles are held in place by different ligaments and controlled to some extent by two muscles: the tensor tympani and stapedius.

A disease state that can significantly impair transmission of sound *via* the ossicles is otitis media which is inflammation of the middle ear mucosa. Acute infection can lead to severe complications such as tympanic membrane perforation, meningitis, subperiosteal abscess, intracranial abscess, sigmoid sinus thrombosis, and mastoiditis. The mastoid is a collection of bony sinuses located behind the ear that are lined by mucosa and connected to the middle ear space *via* the aditus ad antrum. Therefore, all middle ear infections can potentially lead to fluid collecting into the mastoid bone. However, it is when the mastoid bone is infected with bony destruction and abscess that the patient has clinical otomastoiditis.

## INNER EAR

The inner ear consists of the cochlea, vestibular organs, endolymphatic sac and duct. These structures are involved with hearing and balance. The inner ear is housed in the temporal bone. In trauma situations, suspected fracture of the temporal bone should exclude involvement of these inner ear structures and subsequently make sure the cochlea is not involved. Involvement of the cochlea may lead to sensorineural hearing loss. Temporal bone fractures can also lead to possible facial nerve paralysis.

Many medications such as diuretics, aminoglycosides, salicylates and chemotherapeutic agents may cause damage to the hair cells of the cochlea and can be ototoxic and vestibulotoxic.

## EXTERNAL NOSE

The nose plays a prominent role in breathing, olfaction, and humidifying and cleaning the air we breathe. The bony framework of the external nose consists of paired nasal bones attached laterally to the frontonasal process of the maxilla. Inferior to the nasal bones are nasal cartilages and connective tissue with specific relationships that dictate the shape and projection of the nose. Alterations in these relationships by congenital malformations, trauma, inflammatory or infectious disease compromise breathing and may lead to cosmetic deformity.

Congenital malformations of the external nasal framework are rare. A unilateral nasal mass must be imaged to evaluate for intracranial connection prior to removal or biopsy due to possible intracranial complications. An encephalocele represents extracranial herniation of intracranial contents through a defect in the skull. Congenital encephaloceles may be seen as midline nasal masses. Incidence varies by region but ranges from 1 in 3000 to 1 in 30,000 [1, 2]. However, 40% of patients have associated congenital anomalies such as hydrocephalus and agenesis of the corpus callosum. By definition, 100% of encephaloceles contain brain tissue and must be handled with care. Encephaloceles may manifest as pulsatile, soft, bluish compressible masses in the glabella region or on the nasal dorsum. They may also present as intranasal masses. They can enlarge with crying or compression of the jugular veins. Once suspected, a high resolution computed tomography (CT) or magnetic resonance imaging (MRI) should be obtained to define anatomy and identify associated malformations. A lesion suspected to have intracranial connection should not be biopsied.

Nasal dermoid cysts are noted in infancy and can present anywhere from the glabella to the nasal tip. Gliomas present after birth and represent extracranial glial tissue but may have some intracranial connection. Both gliomas and dermoid cysts may have intracranial connections and need further evaluation prior to surgical treatment.

Infantile hemangioma (IH) is the most common tumors of infancy, occurring in 5-10% of all infants [3]. Caucasian females with a history of prematurity are at greatest risk. Cutaneous IH may occur anywhere on the body but over 60% occur on the head and neck. IH may be present initial as pale flat areas but then proliferate into cherry red raised lesions that are expected to involute within 12 months. Treatment is typically monitoring disease unless there is a functional deficit such as vision or hearing compromise, bleeding or ulceration, or a high volume cardiac shunting. Medical therapy includes use of topical, intralesional or systemic corticosteroids, chemotherapy and recently beta blockade. Failure of medical management may require surgical intervention

## INTERNAL NOSE AND NASAL CAVITY

The internal nose comprises of two nasal cavities extending from the both nares to the choanae. The nasal septum divides the nose into two sides. The nasal septum consists of cartilage and bone. Relevant pathologies of the nasal septum include rhinitis, epistaxis, septal abscess, septal hematoma and septal masses.

Epistaxis is a common pediatric complaint with a majority stemming from anterior sources. Approximately 80% of epistaxis occurs in the anterior region of the nasal septum. The nose and sinus arterial blood supply come from both the external and internal carotid arteries. Bleeding from arterial sources is usually localized to the area supplied by the anterior ethmoid artery, superior labial artery, greater palatine artery, and branches of the sphenopalatine artery (Kiesselbach's plexus). Most epistaxis can be controlled by external pressure and topical vasoconstrictor sprays, while the primary etiology of epistaxis is addressed. Epistaxis recalcitrant to external pressure and vasconstrictors may be stopped by nasal packing, cautery, embolizationand and endoscopic sinus surgery. Chemical or electrical nasal cautery performed bilaterally can potentially lead too septal perforation, caution is advised.

Septal hematoma may be caused by blunt and/or penetrating trauma. It represents collection of blood underneath the perichondrium and effectively separating the quadrangular cartilage from its blood supply. When diagnosed, these should be drained and packed as failure to do so may result in cartilage damage and a saddle nose deformity. Septal abscess is accumulation of infected purulent material underneath the mucoperichondrium. This should be drained and treated with antibiotics targeting *Staphylococcus aureus.*

Approximately 90% of nasal airway flows along the floor of the nasal cavity. Nasal airway obstruction may be caused by congenital anomalies, septal deviation, inferior turbinate hypertrophy and adenoid hypertrophy. The nasal septal deviation can cause nasal airway obstruction. If this occurs secondary to early birth trauma, it may need early intervention as neonates are preferentially nasal breathers for the first 6 weeks of life. In adolescence, septoplasty can be performed but intervention too early can affect midfacial growth.

Nasal obstruction may be secondary to edema of the nasal mucosa from inflammation or hypertrophy of the inferior turbinates. The inferior turbinates serve to humidify and clean our nasal airflow. Allergic rhinitis may contribute to the turbinate hypertrophy; therefore, intranasal topical steroids may be helpful. Failure of medical improvement is an indication of surgical reduction of the inferior turbinates.

Adenoid hypertrophy is an overgrowth of lymphatic tissue that lies in the posterior nasopharynx. Hypertrophy of the adenoids can lead to nasal airway obstruction and also decrease posterior nasal drainage. This obstruction can lead to recurrent sinus infections. Removal of the adenoids can improve sinus infections in 50% of the cases [4]. Adenoid removal is also considered for upper airway obstruction and for recurrent ear infections on the placement of a second pair of ear tubes. Without surgical intervention, the adenoid pad will regress during the time of puberty in most children.

Congenital pyriform aperture stenosis (CPAS) is caused by overgrowth of the nasal process of the maxilla. The symptom complex is variable and may consist of cyclical cyanosis and respiratory distress. CPAS is diagnosed by clinical exam and confirmed by high resolution, fine cut computed tomography scan [5]. It is associated with other congenital anomalies such as a single central incisor, pituitary abnormalities, absence of the corpus callosum, and holoprosencephaly.

Congenital choanal atresia/stenosis occurs in 1 per 5000 live births [6]. It is twice as common in female patients and also more likely to be unilateral (~60% right side dominance). It is caused by failure of resorption of the nasobuccal membrane. Anatomically, it is actual blockage of the nasal cavity (typically posterior nasal cavity) by tissue typically consists of bony-membranous components. Symptoms include cyclical cyanosis, unilateral rhinorrhea, and nasal obstruction. Children with bilateral choanal stenosis may have pronounced cyanosis with feeding. Diagnosis consists of classic inability to pass a 6 french nasal catheter, and is confirmed by nasal endoscopy and imaging (CT). Oral airway is a simple, temporary measure for neonates with choanal atresia and life threatening cyanosis. Bilateral stenosis may require repair within the first few weeks of life while unilateral stenosis may be repaired electively later in life. Patients with choanal atresia may have a CHARGE association (Coloboma of the retina, Heart defects, Atresia choanae, Retardation of growth, Genitourinary anomalies, Ear abnormalities) and should be examined properly for these associations.

Nasal polyps (NP) are the most common benign inflammatory masses of the nasal cavity. They are seen as translucent, smooth masses which can originate anywhere in the nasal cavity and even protrude into the anterior and posterior nasal cavity. Symptomatic patients with NP complain of nasal obstruction, sinusitis, facial pressure or pain, and decreased smell. Children with nasal polyps should undergo screening for cystic fibrosis due to the high prevalence of NP in children with cystic fibrosis.

## PARANASAL SINUSES

There are four pairs of paranasal sinuses: the maxillary, ethmoid, frontal and sphenoid sinuses. The maxillary sinuses are the first pair of sinuses to develop in utero and continue to grow through the teenage years. They are located in the body of the maxilla and bounded superiorly by the floor or of the orbit, anteriorly by the canine fossa, and inferiorly by the alveolar process of the maxilla. Ethmoid sinuses are present at birth and reach adult size by age 12. They are bounded superiorly by the skull base and laterally by the thin lamina papyracea or medial wall of the orbits. The sphenoid sinuses are minimal at birth and are not well pnuematized in a neonate. They reach adult size between ages 12-15 years. Sphenoid sinuses are located in the sphenoid bone and are surrounded by several vital structures: the pituitary superiorly, and critical neurovascular structures laterally (the carotid artery, optic nerve, cavernous sinus, third to sixth cranial nerves). The frontal sinuses are not present at birth and continue to develop even through the end of the second decade.

Because of the proximity of the orbit and intracranial cavity to the sinuses, acute rhinosinusitis can lead to preseptal cellulitis of the orbit, which clinically manifests as periorbital edema, pain and erythema. Vision is not compromised and there is no eye movement restriction. Treatment is primarily medical with intravenous antibiotics and supportive care. Orbital cellulitis is spread of disease beyond the orbital septum. Patients with this level of complication have proptosis, impairment of vision and may have limitation of extraocular muscle movement. In more severe cases, subperiosteal abscess (SPA), or collection of pus between the orbital periosteum and bone, may occur. In SPA, there is proptosis, gaze restriction, reduction of visual acuity and evidence of abscess formation on CT or magnetic resonance imaging (MRI). Orbital abscess represents accumulation of pus within the orbit and requires immediate surgical drainage. Finally, cavernous sinus thrombosis may occur as a result of spread of infection beyond the orbit, into the cavernous sinus. This is a serious complication manifested by severe proptosis, vision loss, opthalmoplegia, and evidence of toxicity. Due to the serious nature of these complications, urgent medical management and possible surgical evaluation is necessary. Given the proximity of the paranasal sinuses to intracranial anatomy, there may also be intracranial complications of acute rhinosinusitis. These include meningitis, epidural abscess, subdural abscess, and brain abscess.

## THE NECK

From superficial to deep, the neck has many layers where clinical correlation is relevant. An understanding about the depth of anatomy will provide knowledge of the pathophysiology of head and neck disease.

Anterior Triangle: The anterior triangle of the neck encompasses a triangle formed by the anterior border of the sternocleidomastoid muscle (SCM), the jaw or body of the mandible, and the midline of the neck defined by the trachea or windpipe. Within this triangle lie essential nerves, muscles, glands, cartilage, bones, arteries, veins, and lymphatics of the head and neck.

Just anterior to the midpoint of the SCM lies the palpable pulse of the carotid artery. The common carotid artery branches into the external and internal carotid artery. The internal carotid artery's first branch is the ophthalmic artery before it enters into the intracranial cavity. The external carotid has many branches that supply the thyroid gland, the tongue, and the remainder of the head and neck.

The internal jugular vein lies just lateral to the carotid artery within the vascular sheath. In thin individuals the jugular pulsations or the external branches of the jugular vein are visible in the anterior neck.

Running tangentially to the jugular vein are the deep cervical lymph nodes. The nasopharynx and pharynx drain directly to the deep cervical nodes. Particularly the tonsils drain through the parapharyngeal space into the deep cervical nodes. Therefore, many infections from the nasopharynx, oropharynx, and hypopharynx will drain to the deep cervical nodes and lead to infectious lymphadenitis. As lymph nodes enlarge with infection, there may be central necrosis and suppurative lymphadenitis. Suppurative lymphadenitis requires antibiotic and possible surgical drainage in cases.

The submandibular gland lies in the superior portion of the anterior triangle of the neck, and is palpable in most children. Adjacent to the submandibular gland are the deep cervical nodes, the jugular vein, internal carotid artery, the submandibular salivary duct and the lingual and hypoglossal nerves.

Many structures in the head and neck developed from the embryonal branchial arches. Aberrations in branchial arch development may lead to congenital anomalies. Branchial abnormalities may be categorized into branchial cysts, sinuses, or a fistula. A cyst has no communication to a body surface, the sinus has a single communication to surface, and a fistula has two communications. Due to embryological development all branchial cleft abnormalities except fourth will be localized in the anterior triangle of the neck, running along the border of the sternocleidomastoid muscle. Fourth branchial abnormalities can be found along the sternum and mediastinum.

First brachial cleft abnormalities are a duplication of portions of the external auditory canal. These may involve the parotid gland, middle ear, and facial nerve. Type I first brachial cysts are located near the external auditory canal. Type II cysts are found in the superior portion of anterior triangle of the neck near the submandibular gland.

Second branchial abnormalities are identified along the anterior border of the upper third of the sternocleidomastoid muscle and adjacent to the muscle. Second branchial abnormalities may be a sinus, cyst, or fistula. A fistula may connect a tract from the skin of the anterior triangle, bifurcating the internal and external carotid artery, and ending into the tonsillar fossa.

Third branchial cleft cysts abnormalities are located along the anterior border of the sternocleidomastoid muscle as well. However, the third branchial fistulas lie posterior to the carotid artery and end in the pharynx at the pyriform sinus by piercing the thyrohyoid membrane.

A fourth branchial abnormality arises from the lateral neck and parallels the course of the recurrent laryngeal nerve, which is around the aorta on the left and around the subclavian artery on the right. The fourth branchial fistulas will end in the pyriform sinus of the pharynx and may present with suppurative infections of the thyroid gland, predominately on the left side. However, fourth branchial abnormalities may also be seen in the mediastinum and sternum.

Another abnormality of the anterior triangle is fibromatosis colli or a pseudotumor of the sternocleidomastoid muscle. This may be related to birth trauma and is clinically evident with mass found along the lower third of the sternocleidomastoid muscle. There may be associated torticollis of the child. These usually appear in the first two months of life and usually resolve with physical therapy. Ultrasound may be useful to define muscular origin of the mass.

The posterior triangle of the neck is bordered by the sternocleidomastoid muscle, the clavicle, and the anterior border of the trapezius. Within the posterior triangle lies the accessory nerve, arterial branches from the thryocervical trunk from the subclavian, cutaneous sensory branches, and lymphatics. Of clinical relevance are the lymphatics of the posterior triangle. These will be the drainage sites for the nasopharynx, ear, and pharynx. Isolated large lesions of the posterior cervical and supraclavicular lymphatics may be suspicious for malignancy.

In the midline of the neck, the trachea and larynx are easily palpable. The cricoid cartilage, which is the only complete tracheal ring, may be the most palpable landmark on a child. Dermoid cysts and thyroglossal duct cysts are the most common lesions along the midline of the neck. A dermoid cyst is lined by ectoderm and can occur anywhere in the head and neck.

A thyroglossal duct cyst is a remnant of the thyroid gland as it descends from its embryologic origin from the foramen cecum of the tongue to its natural position in the lower third of the neck. At the border of the anterior two thirds and the posterior third of the tongue lies the foramen cecum. The endoderm at the foramen cecum descends in the anterior midline neck through the mid-portion of the hyoid bone to its natural position in the lower third of the neck. Because the cyst is attached to the base of tongue, protrusion of the tongue will make the midline neck mass move superiorly and inferiorly. Any remnant of this tract can form a thyroglossal duct cyst. The thyroglossal duct cyst may become infected and require antibiotics and at times drainage. In a small portion of patients the thyroglossal duct cyst may be the only functional thyroid tissue for the child and there is a 1% chance of malignant transformation of these cysts.

## LARYNX

The pediatric larynx functions in coordinating breathing/respiration, phonation, and airway protection with swallowing. Subsequently, dysfunction of the larynx manifest in the form of abnormal breathing, aspiration, and hoarseness.

The larynx is divided into the supraglottis, glottis and subglottis. The glottic larynx consists of the epiglottis, false vocal folds, arytenoids and aryepiglottic folds. The glottis larynx consists primarily of the paired true vocal cords while the subglottis is the anatomy from just below the inferior edge of the true vocal cords to the cricoid ring. These subsites contain different tissues and are made up of cartilage (epiglottis, thyroid, cricoid, paired arytenoid, corniculate and cuneiform), bone (hyoid), muscle and mucosa.

There are two main categories of muscles that are involved in laryngeal function: extrinsic muscles and intrinsic muscles. Extrinsic muscles attach to the laryngeal structures from other surrounding structures. They help to move the larynx up, down or backward. They are geniohyoid, mylohyoid, omohyoid, digastric, sternohyoid and sternothyroid muscles. Intrinsic muscles are located *within* the laryngeal complex and are directly involved in glottal abduction (spread apart) during respiratory tasking or adduction (brought together) during phonation. These include the cricothyroid, lateral cricothyroid, thyroarytenoid, posterior thyroarytenoid, transverse arytenoid and vocalis muscles.

Sensory innervation of the supraglottic and infraglottic larynx is mediated by the recurrent laryngeal nerve and the internal branch of the superior laryngeal nerve respectively. The recurrent laryngeal nerve is also responsible for motor innervation of the intrinsic muscles of the larynx except for the cricothyroid muscle, which is innervated by the external branch of the superior laryngeal nerve. The cricothyroid muscle is involved with increasing the pitch of your voice. Blood supply is provided by the inferior and superior thyroid arteries.

There are some fundamental differences between adult *versus* the pediatric larynx. Awareness of these differences is instrumental in constructing a differential diagnosis of airway diseases and more importantly, in managing airway emergencies [7-9].

The neonatal larynx is more anterior and superior than the adult larynx. Superior margin of the epiglottis is at the level of the first cervical vertebrae (C1)-this is higher than the adult larynx and positioned to approximate the soft palate in infants. In newborn to children age 2 and below, the hyoid bone may be found at C2-C3. This positioning permits simultaneous suckling and breathing. The infant epiglottis is also significantly shorter than the adult epiglottis. The larynx continues to descend with growth with inferior aspect located at C4 at birth, C5 at 2 years, C6 at 5 years and C6-C7 in mid-to-late teenage years. With this descent, the shape also transforms from a conical structure into a cylindrical apparatus.

The size of the infant larynx is a third of the adult larynx. In anterior-posterior dimension, the pediatric larynx is 7mm and lateral dimension is 4mm. The length of the true vocal cord in the infant is 2.5 to 3.0mm while the adult TVC measures 17-21mm.The narrowest portion of the infant larynx is the subglottis. Large airway foreign bodies will lodge in the subglottis because it is the narrowest portion of the airway. Subsequently, cuffed endotracheal tubes or tight fitting tubes may cause edema and future subglottic stenosis. The vocal cord marks the narrowest portion in the adult larynx.

Phonation is controlled by the innervation discussed above and more importantly, vibration of the layers of the true vocal cord from airstream passing through the cords. On gross level, the task of voicing is better understood from the perspective of the Bernoulli's principle in fluid dynamics. In simple terms, as the speed of air passes through the vocal cords, the pressure lowers causing a vacuum effect and leads to vibration of the true vocal folds. The true vocal cords consist of multiple layers with different degrees of elasticity. The external layers have the highest elasticity. When the vocal cords are adducted during phonation, the stream of airflow is stopped by the adducted cords [10, 11].Subglottic pressure builds until it is high enough to push the cords apart. As the airstream passes through this constriction, the pressure drops and this drop subsequently allows adduction of the cords and the cycle repeats. The frequency of each cycle is known as the fundamental frequency and contributes to the perceived pitch. In summary, for adequate phonation and a good cry, the infant needs intact neurological control of the vocal cords, sufficient expiratory volume to provide good airstream and good elasticity of the true vocal cord layers.

Stridor is the audible, high pitched sound caused by turbulent air flow passing by a fixed or variable obstruction. The obstruction may occur at the vocal cords or above or below the cords. It may or may not be associated with respiratory distress. In the context of the respiratory cycle, stridor maybe inspiratory, expiratory or biphasic. Inspiratory stridor suggests supraglottic obstruction, while expiratory stridor may clue the practioneer to investigate the tracheobronchial airway. Biphasic stridor may be secondary to subglottic or glottis obstruction [12, 13]. Stertor is a deep, sonorous sound that typically occurs in sleep and less frequently in the awake patient. It can be seen in children with upper airway obstruction, hypotonia or with poor neuromuscular control. Stertor may also result from air. Wheezing is not caused by laryngeal pathology and indicates lower airway issues.

Laryngomalacia is the most common congenital abnormality of the larynx and the most common cause of stridor in infants. The etiology of the disorder is not entirely understood but poor laryngeal tone due to altered sensorimotor integration of the brainstem and peripheral reflexes is thought to play a role [14]. 75% of children seen with inspiratory stridor is secondary to laryngomalacia, and most children outgrow the condition with only 10-20% of children requiring surgical intervention [15]. While a majority of inspiratory stridor is laryngomalacia, a flexible fiberoptic laryngoscopy is the key to diagnosis and to eliminate other etiologies of stridor such as vallecular cyst, vocal cord paralysis, saccular cysts, and recurrent respiratory papillomas. The pathophysiology of the inspiratory stridor and obstruction stems from the prolapse of supraglottic tissue during inspiration. This is due to the characteristic laryngeal anatomy of patients with laryngomalacia characterized by shortened aryepiglottic folds and redundant arytenoid mucosa. Obstructive sleep apnea, dysphagia with failure to thrive, cor pulmonale, heart failure, cyanosis, or pectus excavatum are indications for surgery [16]. The prognosis of laryngomalacia is good with 75% of children having spontaneous resolution of symptoms by 18 months of age. 18% of children with laryngomalacia will also have a synchronous airway lesion, which may need to be evaluated by the otolaryngologist [17]. While a majority of cases of laryngomalacia are in newborns, there are a few cases with older children with poor neurologic tone or exercise induced laryngomalacia who may benefit from an otolaryngology evaluation.

Vocal cord paralysis is a common cause of inspiratory or biphasic neonatal stridor and may be unilateral or bilateral in nature. Common etiologies for vocal cord paralysis are idiopathic, secondary to surgery near the vagus or recurrent laryngeal nerves, birth trauma, intracranial lesions, and neurologic disease. The management and treatment of children with unilateral vocal cord paralysis is to balance breathing, aspiration, feeding, and voice. In some cases recovery of vocal cord function is possible, such as following cardiac surgery, which has a 35% rate of spontaneous recovery [18]. Bilateral vocal cord paralysis can occur with severe dyspnea symptoms and may require a tracheotomy. Idiopathic vocal cord paralysis requires imaging from the skull base to the aortic arch to rule out an etiology such as a heart defect or Arnold chiari malformation.

Laryngeal web may present with stridor, hoarseness, and airway obstruction. A laryngeal web can vary in severity of obstruction with a complete laryngeal web being laryngeal atresia, which is only compatible with life following a tracheotomy. Laryngeal webs may also occur with narrowing of the subglottis of the trachea. Genetic consultation should be considered following the diagnosis to look for other comorbidities. Surgical intervention is the treatment for laryngeal webs.

Vallecular cyst is an epithelium lined cyst found at the base of the tongue. It may present with feeding difficulties, failure to thrive, dyspnea, and acute life threatening events. Because of the potential for airway obstruction early surgical intervention is the standard of treatment.

Saccular cysts occur in the ventricle between the true and false vocal cords. The may present with stridor, respiratory distress, hoarseness, or feeding difficulties. Because of possibility of airway obstruction early surgical intervention may be necessary.

Laryngeal clefts are secondary to a failure of fusion and development of the cricoid cartilage and the trachea esophageal septum. A laryngeal cleft can extend to the top of the cricoid cartilage to more inferiorly to the cervical or thoracic trachea. Presenting symptoms range from stridor, cough, feeding difficulties, aspiration, and life threatening cyanosis. Depending on the severity of the cleft and symptoms of the child, the role of surgical management can vary.

Vocal cord nodules, polyps, and cysts are laryngeal lesions that are common causes for hoarseness in children. A common cause for vocal cord nodules and polyps are screaming and yelling by children. Medical and speech therapy is the primary form of treatment for these lesions and surgery is reserved after failing non-surgical therapy. Nodules and polyps respond well to conservative management, but vocal cysts typically do not.

Recurrent respiratory papillomatosis can be a cause for hoarseness, stridor, or respiratory distress in children. Papillomas are benign growths caused by the human papilloma virus. Most children are diagnosed early in childhood and there is a small potential for malignant transformation of these papillomas. Papillomas can occur anywhere along the respiratory tract and aggressive surgical therapy is the primary form of treatment.

## ORAL CAVITY AND OROPHARYNX

The oral cavity and oropharynx extends from the vermillion border of the lips to the posterior pharyngeal wall. Within this cavity are many structures such as our tongue, teeth, and tonsils. Our primary dentition of twenty primary teeth erupts beginning at 8 months. By age six our permanent teeth begin erupting and by age thirteen all of our primary teeth have been replaced. As an adult we have 32 teeth. Behind our lower central incisors, lies the Wharton's duct, which drains the salivary secretions of the sublingual and submandibular gland.

Also in this floor of mouth can lie an abnormally tight lingual frenulum, which is called ankyloglossia or tongue tie. This short lingual frenulum attaching to the tongue tip and causing a heart shaped tongue can lead to difficulty of latching for breast feeding, difficulty lifting the tongue to the palate, impaired side to side movement, and difficult with tongue protrusion. Indication for a lingual frenotomy for ankyloglossia include breastfeeding difficulty, articulation problems, psychologic problems, and periodontal disease.

Innervated by the hypoglossal and lingual nerve, the tongue is essential organ for swallowing, articulation, taste, and breathing. Many lesions can be seen on the tongue including, ulcers, leukoplakia, mucoceles, and infectious lesions. As discussed earlier, the thyroid gland begins at the foramen cecum of the tongue, and lingual thyroid may be present at the base of tongue.

The parotid gland which lies anterior to the ear canal bilaterally contains the salivary gland tissue and the facial nerve. The parotid glands provide a majority of our salivary secretions during mastication. Stenson's duct drains the salivary secretions of the parotid gland and its opening is opposite the upper second molar.

Cleft lip is classified as unilateral or bilateral and as complete or incomplete. A complete cleft involves the entire upper lip, and is often associated with an alveolar cleft. An incomplete cleft lip only involves a portion of the lip. Unilateral *versus* bilateral refers to which side or both of the lip.

Cleft Palates are classified as unilateral or bilateral and as complete or incomplete. In addition, cleft palates are classified according to their location relative to the incisive foramen. Clefts of the primary palate occur anterior to the incisive foramen, and clefts of the secondary palate involve the segment posterior to the incisive foramen [19]. A unilateral cleft of the secondary palate is defined by a cleft in which the palatal process of the maxilla on one side is fused with the nasal septum A bilateral complete cleft of the secondary palate has no point of fusion between the maxilla and the nasal septum. A complete cleft of the entire palate involves both the primary and secondary palate, including one or both sides of the premaxilla/alveolar arch, and frequently involves a cleft lip. The least severe incomplete cleft is the submucous cleft palate (SMCP) in which the underlying palatal musculature is deficient and inappropriately attached. Associated features include a bifid uvula, a zona pellucida (bluish midline region representing the muscle deficiency), and a notch in the posterior hard palate.

The tonsils are lymphatic tissue that screens infections as they enter or aerodigestive system. They lie within the tonsillar fossa created by a pocket formed by the anterior and posterior pillar, which lie on either side of the soft palate and uvula. Tonsils are graded from 1+ to 4+ [20]. Tonsils that lie from lateral to medial and obstruct 25% of the oropharyngeal airway are 1+ in size, 50% are 2+, 75% are 3+, and 100% or kissing tonsils are 4+ in size.

Clinical practice guidelines recommend tonsillectomy for sleep disordered breathing with history or polysomnogram suggesting obstructive sleep apnea. Tonsillectomy for recurrent throat infection is recommended with a frequency of at least 7 episodes in the past year, or at least 5 episodes per year for 2 years, or at least 3 episodes per year for 3 years with documentation in the medical record for each episode of sore throat and one or more of the following: temperature >38.3°C, cervical adenopathy, tonsillar exudate, or positive test for GABHS. Modifying factors for tonsillectomy are multiple antibiotic allergy/intolerance, PFAPA (periodic fever, aphthous stomatitis, pharyngitis, and adenitis), or history of peritonsillar abscess [21].

Lying lateral to the tonsils are the palatoglossus and palatopharyngeus muscle. The space between the tonsillar capsule and the muscles is the peritonsillar space. Tonsillitis can lead to the formation of purulence and form a peritonsillar abscess. Symptomatically these patients can have odyntophagia, drooling, a hot potato voice, and at times otalgia and trismus. Trismus is secondary to inflammation caused near the muscles of mastication.

Infection of the tonsil or a peritonsillar abscess can lead to spread of infection to the parapharyngeal space. The parapharyngeal space is a pyramidal space going from the skull base to the hyoid bone of the neck. Infections of the parapharyngeal space can lead to jugulodigastric lymphadenitis. Infections can potentially spread along the vascular sheath toward the mediastinum.

Parapharyngeal infections may also enter into the retropharyngeal space as well. The retropharyngeal space lies between the buccopharyngeal fascia, which lies under the pharyngeal mucosa, and the alar fascia. The retropharyngeal begins at the skull base and extends to the mediastinum to the level of the carina. The retropharygeal lymph nodes drain infections from the nose, sinuses, and throat. These infections usually occur in young children and present with fever, dysphagia, drooling, neck pain and stiffness, and cervical lymphadenitis. Retropharyngeal space infections can also enter posteriorly into the danger space, which lies between the alar fascia and prevertebral fascia, and into the prevertebral space which lies behind the danger space. The danger space can extend to the mediastinum to the level of the diaphragm and the prevertebral space can extend to the abdominal cavity.

Therefore, due to the possible connections of the head and neck spaces, a peritonsillar abscess can potentially lead to a retropharyngeal abscess that can be progress to life threatening mediastinitis [22].

## ACKNOWLEDGEMENT

None Declared.

## CONFLICT ON INTEREST

The authors declare that there are no conflict of interest.

## REFERENCES

[1]     Connor SE. Imaging of skull-base cephalocoeles and cerebrospinal fluid leaks. Clin Radiol. 2010 Oct;65(10):832-41.

[2]     Ravindhra G. Elluru, Christopher T. Wootten. Congenital Malformations of the Nose. Cummings CW, ed. Cummings Otolaryngology-Head and Neck Surgery. 5th ed. Philadelphia: Mosby Elsevier; 2010. Pp 2686-2697

[3]     Holland KE, Drolet BA. Infantile hemangioma. Pediatr Clin North Am. 2010 Oct; 57(5):1069-83. Epub 2010 Aug 21

[4]     Vandenberg SJ, Heatley DG. Efficacy of adenoidectomy in relieving symptoms of chronic sinusitis in children. *Arch Otolaryngol Head Neck Surg.* 1997;123(7):675-678

[5]     Brown OE, Myer CM 3rd, Manning SC. Congenital nasal pyriform aperture stenosis, Laryngoscope. 1989 Jan;99(1):86-91.

[6]     Corrales CE, Koltai PJ. Choanal atresia: current concepts and controversies. Curr Opin Otolaryngol Head Neck Surg. 2009 Dec;17(6):466-70.

[7]     Sapienza CM, Ruddy BH, Baker S. Laryngeal structure and function in the pediatric larynx: clinical applications. Lang Speech Hear Serv Sch. 2004 Oct;35(4):299-307.

[8]     Hudgins PA, Siegel J, Jacobs I, Abramowsky CR. The normal pediatric larynx on CT and MR.AJNR Am J Neuroradiol. 1997 Feb;18(2):239-45.

[9]     Cotton RT. Management and prevention of subglottic stenosis in infants and children. In: Bluestone CD, Stool SE, Kenna MA, eds. Pediatric Otolaryngology. 3rd ed. Philadelphia, Pa: Saunders; 1996:1373–1389

[10]   Timcke R, Von Ledgen H, Moore P. Laryngeal vibrations: measurements of the glottic wave. II. Physiologic variations. AMA Arch Otolaryngol. 1959 Apr;69(4):438-44

[11]    Benninger MS, Alessi D, Archer S, Bastian R, Ford C, Koufman J, Sataloff RT, Spiegel JR, Woo P. Vocal foldscarring: currentconcepts and management. Otolaryngol Head Neck Surg. 1996 Nov;115(5):474-82.

[12]    Leung AK, Cho H. Diagnosis of stridor in children.Am Fam Physician. 1999 Nov 15;60(8):2289-96.

[13]    Boudewyns A, Claes J, Van de Heyning P. Clinical practice: an approach to stridor in infants and children.Eur J Pediatr. 2010 Feb;169(2):135-41.

[14]    Thompson DM. Abnormal sensorimotor integrative function of the larynx in congenital laryngomalacia; a new theory of etiology. Laryngoscope 2007; 117 (suppl 114):1-33.

[15]    Olney DR, Greinwald JH Jr, Smith RJ, Bauman NM. Laryngomalacia and its treatment. Laryngoscope. 1999 Nov; 109 (11): 1770-5.

[16]    Denoyelle, F, Mondain, M. Gresillon, N et al. Failure and compications of suprglottoplasty in children. Archives of otolaryngology and head and neck surgery 2003:129(10):1077-1080

[17]    Mancuso RF, Choi SS, Zalzal GH, Grundfast KM, Laryngomalacia. The search for the second lesion.Arch Otolaryngol Head Neck Surg. 1996 Mar;122(3):302-6.

[18]    Truong, MT, Messner, AH, Kerschner, JE et Al. Pediatric vocal fold paralysis after cardiac surgery: rate of of recovery and sequelae. Otolaryngology and Head and Neck Surgery 2007:151(3):312-315

[19]    Friedman, O, Wang, T., Milczuk, H. Cleft Lip and Palate. Cummings Otolaryngology-Head and Neck Surgery. 5th ed. Philadelphia: Mosby Elsevier; 2010. Pp 2659-2676

[20]    Brodsky L. Modern assessment of tonsils and adenoids. *Pediatr Clin North Am.* 1989;36(6):1551-1569

[21]    Baugh RF, et al. Clinical practice guideline: tonsillectomy in children. Otolaryngol Head Neck Surg. 2011 Jan;144(1 Suppl):S1-30.)

[22]    Kirse, D. Roberson, DW. Surgical management of retropharyngeal space infections in children. Laryngoscope 2001 Aug;111(8):1413-22.

Send Orders of Reprints at reprints@benthamscience.net

# CHAPTER 2

## Approach to Pediatric Neck Masses

## Michael E. McCormick[1] and Rahul K. Shah[2*]

[1]*Children's Hospital of Wisconsin, Department of Otolaryngology/Medical College of Wisconsin, Children's Hospital Clinics Building, 9000 West Wisconsin Avenue, Suite 540,P.O BOX 1997, Milwaukee, Wisconsin 53226, USA and* [2]*Children's National Medical Center, George Washington University, 111 Michigan Avenue, NW, Washington, D.C. 20010, USA*

**Abstract:** Pediatric neck masses can be divided into two broad categories: congenital and acquired. The most common congenital neck masses in children are branchial cleft cysts and thyroglossal duct cysts. The majority of pediatric neck masses are acquired and can be sub-classified as either infectious or inflammatory. Commonly encountered benign tumors include hemangiomas and lipomas. Unlike adult neck masses, malignant neoplasms are rare, accounting for only 15% of persistent neck masses. Cervical malignancies in children include rhabdomyosarcoma, lymphoma, and neuroblastoma. A careful history and physical examination is paramount in the diagnostic approach to the pediatric patient with a neck mass. Radiologic and laboratory tests can assist in the diagnosis, and occasionally surgical biopsy is necessary.

**Keywords:** Congenital neck mass, lymphadenopathy, neck abscess, branchial cleft, neoplasm, malignancy.

## HISTORY & PHYSICAL EXAMINATION

In evaluating a child with a neck mass, the first and most important assessment is of the child's airway and breathing status. This can usually be determined as soon as the clinician enters the room: a happy, playful child who is singing to his mother does not likely have an impending airway compromise. On the other hand, a stridulous child who is clinging to his parent may be developing obstruction of his airway and requires emergent otolaryngologic evaluation. The other important

*Address correspondence to Rahul K. Shah:** Children's National Medical Center, 111 Michigan Avenue, NW, Washington, D.C. 20010, USA; Tel: 202 476-3712; Fax: 202 476-5038; E-mail: Rshah@cnmc.org

consideration when evaluating these children is whether the child requires inpatient admission.

History alone can often narrow the differential diagnosis substantially, particularly the temporal course and pattern of growth of the neck mass. Infectious lymphadenopathy and abscesses often have a rapid, painful unilateral swelling that follows an upper respiratory infection, while lymphomas and thyroid neoplasms tend to have a more indolent, painless growth pattern. Other key considerations include animal bites or scratches, and preceding trauma to the area. Changes in size with various activities could suggest a particular diagnosis, such as a laryngocele (straining, coughing) or a hemangioma (crying). Finally, the astute clinician can gain useful knowledge from a thorough review of systems, especially in the presence of fatigue, fevers, weight loss, or night sweats [1-2].

A complete head and neck examination is necessary in the evaluation of a child with a neck mass when possible, with particular attention to the size, location, and nature of the neck mass. Children of all ages frequently have benign lymphoid hyperplasia, particularly in the jugulodigastric region posterior to the angle of the mandible, but all lymph nodes >2cm warrant closer investigation. Location alone can help the clinician narrow their differential diagnostic considerations. Common midline lesions include thyroglossal duct cysts and dermoids, while infectious lymhadenopathy, abscesses, and branchial cleft anomalies are more common in the lateral neck. When assessing the nature of the neck mass, consideration should be given to the consistency and mobility. Soft, mobile neck masses are typically cysts or abscesses, while malignancies tend be firmer and fixed to surrounding structures.

Otologic examination can reveal evidence of otomastoiditis in the case of a Bezold's abscess. Nasal examination may demonstrate purulence or nasal masses or decreased nasal airflow. Examination of the mouth and throat should include the floor of mouth, the tonsils, and posterior pharyngeal wall, when visualized. While most diagnoses can be reached with attention given only to the head and neck, it cannot be forgotten that clues can occasionally be found elsewhere on the body, such as axillary or groin lymphadenopathy and cutaneous lesions such as hemangiomas.

## ANCILLARY TESTS

Ultrasound has great utility in the differentiation of solid and cystic masses, and Doppler examination of blood flow can help identify hemangiomas and vascular malformations. Ultrasound is particularly useful in the workup of thyroid masses and in the evaluation of normal thyroid tissue in patients with thyroglossal duct cysts. Its effectiveness requires a skilled technician and is variable between technicians and institutions.

Computed tomography (CT) provides information on the relationship of the neck mass to surrounding structures, such as large blood vessels, bony structures, and the airway. It is helpful in delineating infectious processes in the deep cervical spaces, especially if surgical intervention is anticipated. CT scans do carry the risk of exposing the child to radiation, although current techniques employ faster scans with lower radiation doses.

Magnetic resonance imaging (MRI) provides even better detail in identification of neck masses and is very useful in vascular and lymphatic malformations and certain soft tissue tumors. It avoids the risk of radiation to the child, but usually requires sedation or general anesthesia because of the time required where the child cannot move.

Common laboratory tests utilized in the workup of a child with a neck mass include complete blood count (CBC) with differential, erythrocyte sedimentation rate (ESR), and serologic titer testing (EBV, CMV, HIV, *Bartonella henselae*). A purified protein derivative (PPD) tuberculin test may also be indicated, especially if there is a history of travel to an area where tuberculosis is endemic.

Biopsy of a neck mass is generally reserved for those that do not respond to antibiotics or in certain cases with high suspicion for a neoplastic process. Fine needle aspiration (FNA) biopsy is usually done under ultrasound-guidance and is especially useful for thyroid lesions. FNA can help direct antibiotic therapy by providing cultures in certain infectious processes that do not respond to first-line antibiotics. Open surgical biopsy should be performed by a trained head and neck surgeon and requires general anesthesia in younger children. In cases suspicious for lymphoma, open biopsy provides tissue for complete analysis, including immunohistochemical staining.

## CONGENITAL NECK MASSES

**Branchial cleft cysts** are the most common congenital lesion of the head and neck and are the result of failure of embryonic clefts to completely obliterate during development. Branchial cleft sinuses and fistulas are anomalies with openings to the skin and/or aerodigestive tract. These lesions typically present as nontender, fluctuant masses that may become inflamed during or after an upper respiratory infection. They are often misdiagnosed as an abscess and treated with incision and drainage, and a recurrent cystic neck mass despite surgical drainage is a common presentation of branchial cleft cysts [3-4].

First branchial cleft anomalies are divided into type I and type II. Type I first branchial cleft cysts are blind duplications of the external auditory canal that do not involve the facial nerve. Type II first branchial cleft anomalies are more common and present as an infected or draining mass near the angle of the mandible. These lesions have a tract that passes through the parotid gland close to the facial nerve and enters the external auditory canal. Antibiotics are used when these lesions are acutely infected but definitive therapy is surgical excision of the entire tract. Incomplete surgical therapy will lead to recurrence of the disease.

Second branchial cleft anomalies (Fig. **1**) are the most common type and are usually found high and lateral in the neck, anterior to the sternocleidomastoid muscle. These lesions may open to the skin and may have a tract that passes between the external and internal carotid arteries and enters the tonsillar fossa. They are treated in a similar fashion to first branchial cleft anomalies with complete excision of the entire tract.

Third and fourth branchial cleft anomalies are rare and present lower in the neck. They are often intimately related with the glossopharyngeal, vagus, and superior laryngeal nerves, as well as the carotid arteries and the internal jugular vein. Surgical excision is often employed but carries significant morbidity. There is evidence to suggest that these lesions can be treated with needle aspiration of the cyst and cauterization of the internal opening in the piriform sinus if present; this avoids risk of injury to the surrounding nerves and blood vessels (Fig. **2**).

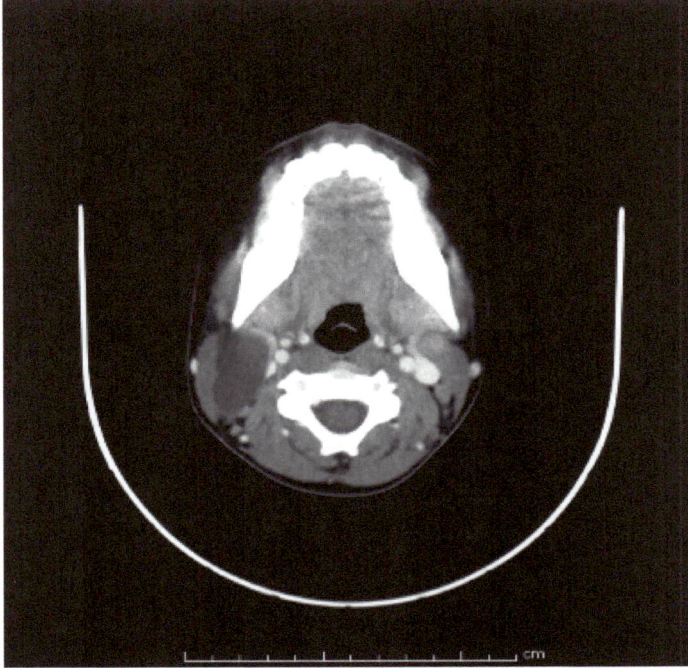

**Figure 1:** CT scan demonstrating right second branchial cleft cyst in a 12 year old child.

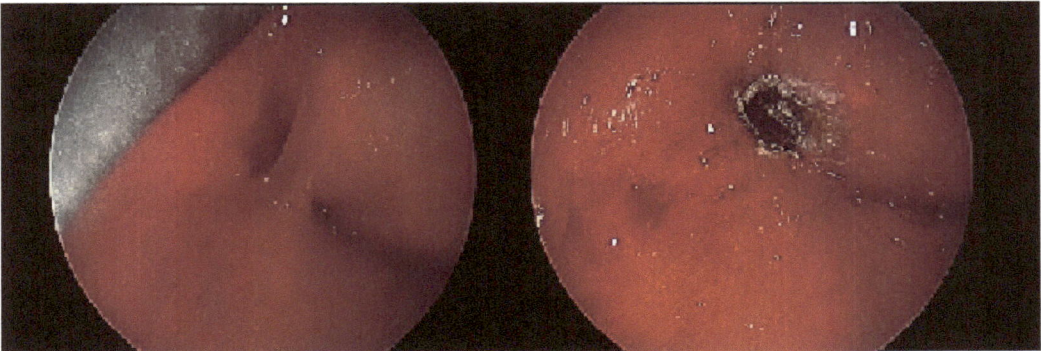

**Figure 2:** Left piriform sinus branchial cleft fistula before (left) and after (right) endoscopic cauterization. This patient had previously undergone incision and drainage of the infected cervical component.

**Thyroglossal duct cysts** are the most common anterior midline neck mass in children, accounting for about one-third of all congenital neck masses. They can form anywhere along the normal tract of descent of the thyroid gland from the foramen cecum in the tongue to its final location in the lower neck, but their most common location is anterior to the hyoid bone (Fig. **3**). The most common presentation is of an asymptomatic mass that moves with swallowing and elevates with tongue protrusion. Thyroglossal duct cysts, like branchial cleft cysts, tend to enlarge with upper respiratory infections. Treatment is surgical excision with removal of the midportion of the hyoid bone (Sistrunk procedure). Proper surgical technique reduces the rate of recurrence from greater than 50% to less than 10%. Prior to surgery, it is essential to establish whether or not the patient has a normal functioning thyroid gland by either ultrasound or thyroid scan [5-6].

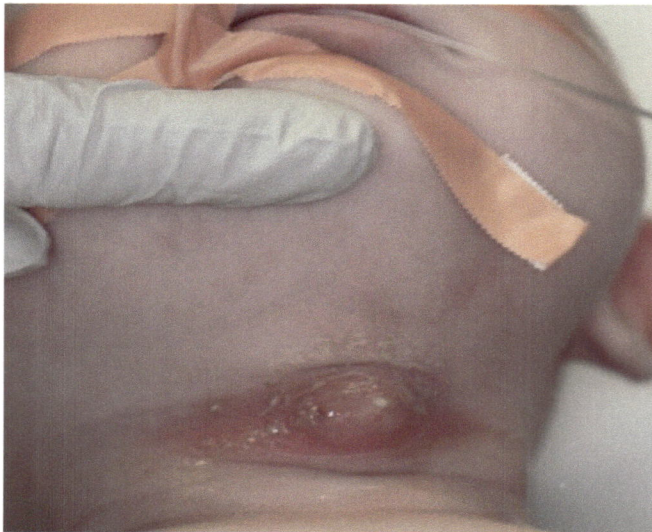

**Figure 3:** Intraoperative photo demonstrating a thyroglossal duct cyst anterior to the hyoid bone.

**Pseudotumor of infancy**, also known as **fibromatosis coli** or **congenital torticollis**, typically appears in the first 1-8 weeks of life as a firm, painless, discrete mass within the sternocleidomastoid muscle. The etiology is unclear, but birth trauma and intrauterine positioning have been suggested as causes for this disease. These masses slowly increase in size in the first 2-3 months, but can usually be managed conservatively with passive and active range of motion exercises. These help prevent future restriction of neck movement. Cases resistant to physiotherapy after 12 months may be treated surgically by dividing the SCM muscle or tendon.

**Lymphatic malformation (LM)** (Fig. **4**) is the current terminology for the previously-termed *lymphangiomas* or *cystic hygromas*, and they are divided into two classes: macrocystic and microcystic. They arise as a maldevelopment of the lymphatic channels that drain the head and neck. LMs usually present in the first year of life as asymptomatic soft, nontender, compressible masses that may enlarge after an upper respiratory infection. They may cause feeding or breathing difficulties depending on their size and location. Imaging with CT and/or MRI is essential in delineating these lesions and how they relate to surrounding structures. Macrocystic lesions can often be treated with needle aspiration and sclerotherapy with agents such as ethanol, OK-432, or doxycycline. Microcystic lesions tend to infiltrate multiple soft tissue structures and are often managed through serial debulkings to improve cosmetic appearances and functional impairments [7].

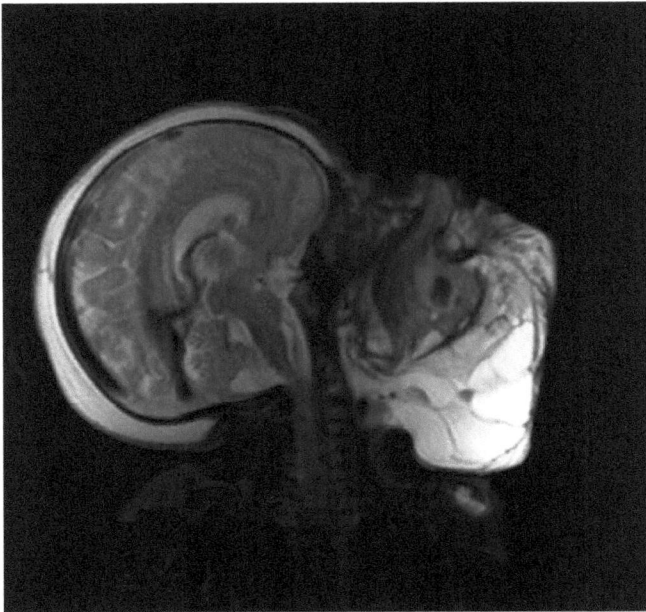

**Figure 4:** MRI of a giant lymphatic malformation causing airway obstruction in a 4 day old. The mass was diagnosed prenatally and an airway was established immediately after delivery *via* an EXIT procedure.

**Hemangiomas** are the most common congenital lesions in the head and neck. They occur most commonly on the skin or mucus membranes, but can occur in deeper tissues such as the parotid gland and the masseter muscle. Hemangiomas of infancy are typically absent at birth but appear within the first few months of life. They tend to proliferate over 6-9 months followed by involution over 2-4 years. Because of their natural course, conservative observation is the recommended treatment, but intervention may be needed if there are complications, such as breathing or feeding difficulty, bleeding, high-output heart failure, or platelet sequestration (Kasabach-Merritt syndrome). Treatment options include surgical excision, medical treatment (systemic corticosteroids and/or propranolol), or laser therapy (for cutaneous lesions).

**Dermoids** and **teratomas** typically develop along embryonic fusion planes. Dermoids consist of epithelium-lined cysts filled with ectodermal and mesodermal elements, while teratomas contain all three germ cell lines. Dermoids most commonly occur in the midline submental area as a nontender mass that does not move with swallowing or tongue protrusion and they are treated with surgical excision. Teratomas are true neoplasms that often present prenatally or at birth as large complex neck masses that can obstruct the airway. Urgent surgical excision is the treatment modality for teratomas of the head and neck [8].

**Ranulas** (Fig. **5**) are thought to occur from obstruction of the sublingual gland's drainage into the floor of the mouth. They are actually not true cysts because they do not have a true epithelial lining, but are actually pseudocysts that fill a connective tissue-lined space. They can occupy the floor of mouth under the tongue, or extend beyond the mylohyoid muscle into the neck (plunging ranula). The diagnosis is usually made clinically and can be confirmed with CT scan. Treatment is surgical and recurrences are common if the sublingual gland is not removed. It is usually not necessary to remove the submandibular gland.

**Foregut duplication cysts** (Fig. **6**) occur at any point along the embryologic foregut, but are most common in the abdomen or thorax. In the head and neck, they are most commonly associated with the tongue. Foregut duplication cysts must have a smooth muscle coat, an epithelial lining representative of the alimentary tract, and an attachment to some portion of the gastrointestinal tract. In the neck, they most commonly present as an asymptomatic mass. Diagnosis is histologic, but suspicion can arise based on CT or MRI findings. Treatment is by complete surgical excision.

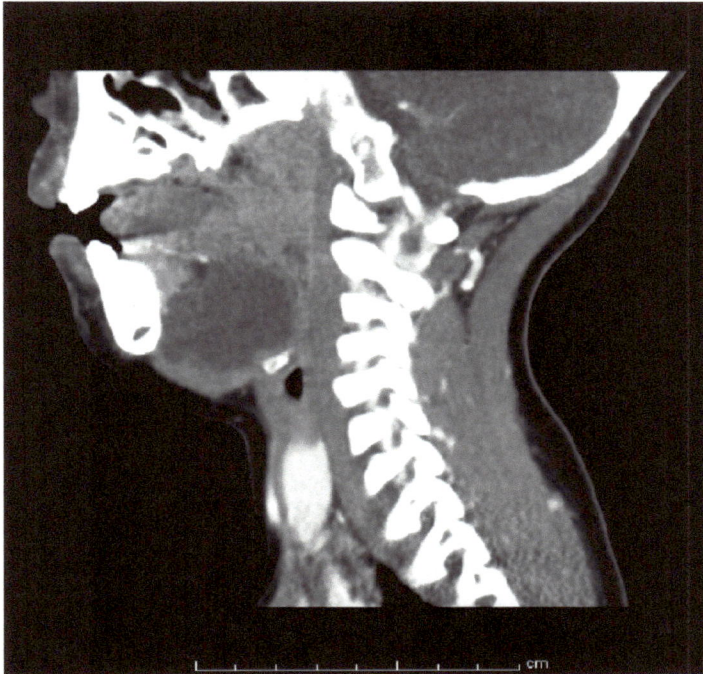

**Figure 5:** Sagittal CT scan of a ranula in a 4 year old female.

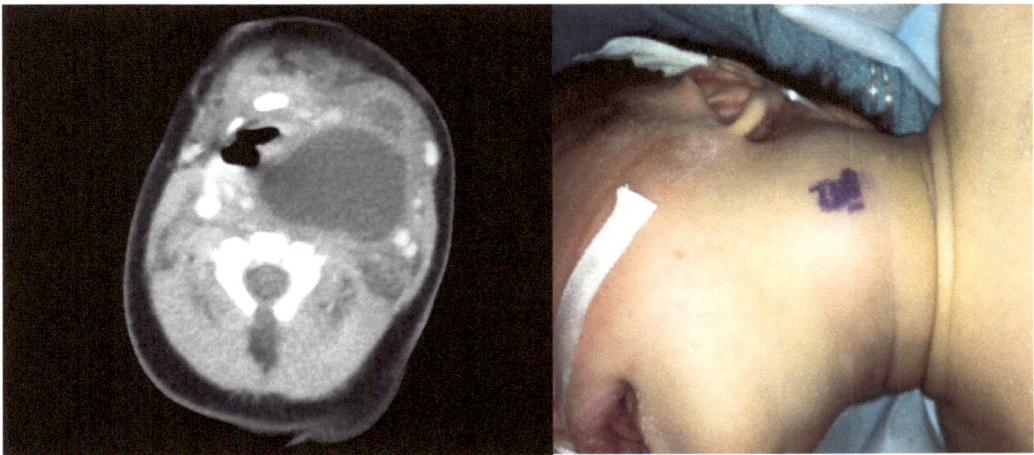

**Figure 6:** CT scan (left) and photo (right) of a 16 day-old with an esophageal duplication cyst.

**Thymic cysts** occur from aberrant implantation of thymic tissue along the path of descent of the thymus to the chest. They are most commonly on the left side of the neck, and cystic in structure and they may enlarge with infections. Thymic cysts can be mistaken for macrocystic LMs on CT or MRI and histologic analysis is required for diagnosis. They are treated with complete surgical excision.

**Laryngoceles** can be congenital or acquired and they may occur in newborns through dilation of the laryngeal saccule into the neck. The presentation is typically a neck mass that enlarges with crying or straining and can be associated with hoarseness or dyspnea. CT is most useful in the diagnosis as it demonstrates the relationship of the mass to the air-filled larynx. The treatment of laryngoceles includes complete surgical excision.

## ACQUIRED INFECTIOUS AND INFLAMMATORY NECK MASSES

**Viral lymphadenopathy** is one of the most common causes of pediatric neck masses, and is usually bilateral and following an upper respiratory infection. Common viral causes of pharyngitis and lymphadenopathy include enterovirus, adenovirus, and coxsackievirus. Epstein-Barr virus (EBV) infections have (usually massive) cervical lymphadenopathy in 93% of children; bilateral posterior cervical lymph node enlargement is most commonly seen with this infection. Other symptoms of EBV include pharyngitis and enlargement of Waldeyer's ring (tonsils and adenoids), as well as generalized lymphadenopathy and splenomegaly. Diagnosis is confirmed with laboratory testing. Cytomegalovirus (CMV) is another virus causing massive cervical lymphadenopathy (75% of cases) and is usually associated with hepatosplenomegaly and rash [9].

Human immunodeficiency virus (HIV) infection can cause cervical lymphadenopathy both directly and indirectly by diminishing the immune system's ability to fight off other viral and bacterial infections. Associated symptoms include weight loss, fatigue, fevers, and hepatosplenomegaly. Suspicion for HIV should be raised in neck masses that fail to respond to antibiotic therapy. Serologic testing is diagnostic. Treatment is with antiretroviral therapy.

**Bacterial lymphadenopathy** is most commonly caused by *Streptococcus pyogenes* or *Staphylococcus aureus*, especially as the incidence of community-acquired methicillin-resistant *S. aureus* (CA-MRSA) increases. The most common presentation is a unilateral neck mass that occurs after an upper respiratory infection and can measure up to 6 centimeters in diameter. Initial management is always with oral antibiotics, but intravenous antibiotics may be needed for more severe cases. Resistance to first-line agents continues to grow and beta-lactamase positive organisms have been reported in up to 34% of cases. An abscess (Fig. **7**) should be suspected when the infection fails to resolve after adequate antibiotic therapy or fluctuance is palpated. Ultrasound can be very useful for distinguishing suppurative and non-suppurative lymphadenopathy and CT scan is sometimes needed for diagnosis. Abscesses are treated with incision and drainage.

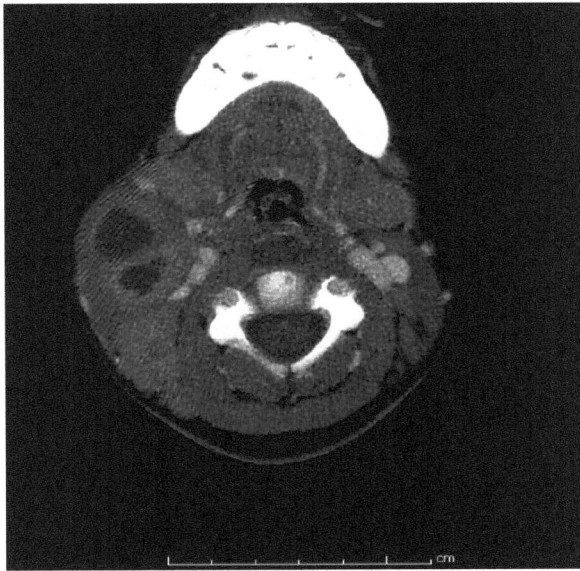

**Figure 7:** Right neck abscess in a 14 month old.

Cervical **mycobacterial infections** are most commonly caused by atypical mycobacteria (59%), usually *M. avium-intracellulare*. However, *M. tuberculosis* accounts for up to 30% of cervical mycobacterial infections and is usually bilateral and associated with pulmonary tuberculosis. Atypical mycobacterial infections present as a unilateral neck mass with overlying skin discoloration. Suspicion should arise with lymphadenopathy resistant to antibiotic therapy, especially in patients who live in or have traveled to endemic areas. Diagnosis is confirmed by placement of a PPD skin test, which is positive in about 95% of cases. Atypical mycobacterial infections tend to have a weaker PPD response, and the diagnosis can remain unclear. Treatment of tuberculous infections is with antituberculous agents. Similarly, atypical mycobacterial infections are usually treated medically as well, but surgical excision is often employed to confirm the diagnosis. Incision and drainage should be avoided because of the risk of chronic fistulization [10].

**Cat-scratch disease** is caused by the gram-negative bacilli *Bartonella henselae*. There is a slight male predominance and >90% of patients have a history of contact with a cat. More than half of patients have axillary lymphadenopathy and most children have fever and malaise. Cultures have poor sensitivity because of the intracellular nature of the organism and the diagnosis is confirmed with serologic tests against the bacterial DNA. The disease is often self-limited, although cat-scratch disease is usually treated with azithromycin. Surgical therapy is rarely indicated [11].

**Kawasaki disease** is a multi organ vasculitis that typically affects children younger than 5 years old. Criteria for diagnosis include fever for 5 days and four of the following: 1) acute cervical lymphadenopathy, 2) erythema and edema of the hands or feet, 3) polymorphous exanthema, usually involving the trunk, 4) bilateral painless conjunctival injection, and 5) lip and oral mucosal changes. Cardiac sequelae include pericardial effusions and coronary artery aneurysms (15-20%). Treatment is with intravenous immunoglobulin (IVIG) and aspirin.

**Sarcoidosis** in children most commonly presents with peripheral lymphadenopathy and cervical nodes are usually discrete, firm, and rubbery. Nonspecific symptoms are common, as is hilar adenopathy. Treatment is usually with corticosteroids. **Rosai-Dorfman disease** is also known as sinus histiocytosis with massive lymphadenopathy. It initially presents with massive bilateral cervical lymph nodes and may involve other nodal groups. Fever and skin nodules may be present as well. Biopsy shows dilated sinuses and numerous plasma cells and histiocytes. Expectant observation usually sees resolution within 6-9 months. Other noninfectious inflammatory disease of the cervical lymph nodes include **Periodic Fevers, Apthous Stomatitis, Pharyngitis, and Adenoiditis (PFAPA)** and **Kikuchi-Fujimoto Disease** [12].

## NEOPLASTIC NECK MASSES

Benign and malignant tumors of the neck are rare in the pediatric population. Two of the more common benign soft tissue tumors in children are lipomas and neurofibromas. **Lipomas** are generally soft and rubbery and grow slowly. **Neurofibromas** typically arise from small cutaneous nerves and may be multiple (neurofibromatosis type I). Both tumors are treated with surgical excision if causing functional or cosmetic disturbances.

The differential diagnosis of a parotid mass in a child differs from that of an adult, and **hemangiomas** are the most common parotid masses in the pediatric patient. However, malignancy is more common in children than in the adult. The most common benign salivary tumor is **pleomorphic adenoma**, which presents as a firm slow-growing mass that does not involve skin or cause facial weakness. Superficial parotidectomy is performed to remove a pleomorphic adenoma. The most common parotid malignancies are **mucoepidermoid** and **acinic cell carcinomas**. These usually present as solitary masses that grow and may cause pain or facial weakness. The treatment and prognosis of each depends on local invasiveness and regional or distant metastatic spread. Most often, superficial parotidectomy is the initial management, with neck dissection and radiation reserved for adjuvant therapies or for recurrence [13].

Thyroid adenomas and carcinomas are rare in the pediatric population. They both usually present as a painless solitary mass in the anterior neck. It is difficult to determine if a thyroid nodule is benign or malignant without FNA biopsy. Therefore, ultrasound-guided biopsy is the first step in the diagnosis of a thyroid nodule. If the diagnosis is still in question, a thyroid scan can be performed, a repeat biopsy can be done at a later date, or a hemithyroidectomy can be performed. The most common thyroid malignancy is **papillary thyroid carcinoma** and it is treated with subtotal or total thyroidectomy. Cervical nodal involvement is common in children (up to 80%) and neck dissection is often required as well. Medical treatment with radioiodine and suppressive thyroid hormone therapy are effective in preventing recurrences.

Lymphomas, both **Hodgkin disease** and **non-Hodgkin's lymphomas (NHL)**, are the most common malignant neoplasm in the neck in children, accounting for about 50% of cervical malignancies. Hodgkin's disease is more common in males and usually presents as an asymptomatic cervical or supraclavicular mass. Constitutional symptoms such as fever, weight loss, or night sweats portend a worse prognosis. Treatment of Hodgkin's involves chemotherapy and/or radiation therapy. Non-Hodgkin's lymphoma usually presents with more disseminated disease and can involve extranodal sites such as the liver, bone marrow, and lung. Chemotherapy is the mainstay of treatment.

**Rhabdomyosarcoma** is the most common soft tissue malignancy in children, and most tumors occur in the head and neck. There are two peak incidences in childhood, between 2-5 years and between 15-19 years, and males are more commonly affected. The most common presentation is a painless, rapidly-enlarging mass that may cause obstruction of the aerodigestive tract. The diagnosis is made by excisional biopsy and treatment is multimodality, with roles for surgery, chemotherapy, and radiation. Prognosis is poor with only 2/3 of patients experiencing long-term survival.

**Neuroblastoma** (Fig. **8**) is the second most common malignant neck mass in children, and the most common in younger children. In the neck, infants will present with a neck mass that can be asymptomatic or can be causing compression of the trachea and/or esophagus. Horner's syndrome may be included in the presentation as well. Diffuse involvement is not uncommon, so evaluation should include imaging of the neck, chest, and abdomen. Management depends on the extent of disease, with surgery reserved for localized disease [14].

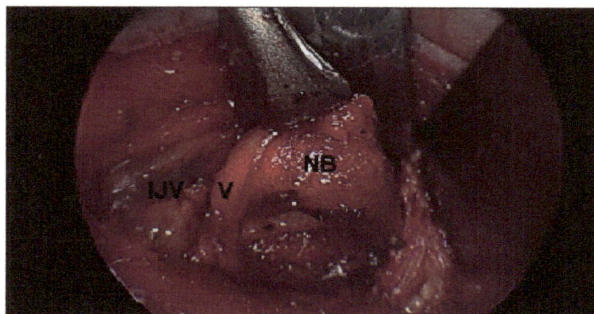

**Figure 8:** Congenital neuroblastoma (NB) of the left cervical sympathetic chain in a 5 month old female. The internal jugular vein (IJV) and vagus nerve (V) are visualized. The child presented with congenital Horner's syndrome and the lesion was discovered on MRI of the neck.

# CONCLUSION

Pediatric neck masses carry an extensive differential diagnosis, which can often be narrowed by a thorough history and physical examination. Radiologic and laboratory studies can assist when the diagnosis is uncertain. Biopsy can be obtained either under image-guidance or by a trained head and neck surgeon. Most neck masses in children are either congenital or inflammatory in nature, and malignancies are rare. The most common congenital lesions are branchial cleft anomalies and thyroglossal duct cysts. Viral or bacterial lymphadenopathy is an extremely common cause of cervical swelling in children, especially in the history of a recent upper respiratory tract infection. Lymphoma is the most common malignant neoplasm found in the neck in children. High suspicion should be raised for malignancy in the context of a large mass that is unresponsive to antibiotics, especially when associated with constitutional symptoms, such as weight loss, fever, or night sweats.

# ACKNOWLEDGEMENT

None declared.

# CONFLICT OF INTEREST

The authors of this chapter have no conflict of interest to declare.

# REFERENCES

[1]     Brown RL and Azizkhan RG. "Pediatric head and neck lesions." *Pediatr Clin North Am.* Aug 1998; 45(4): 889-905.
[2]     Wetmore RF, Potsic WP. "Differential Diagnosis of Neck Masses." In: *Otolaryngology: Head & Neck Surgery, 5th Edition.* Cummings CW *et al.* (Eds). Mosby-Elsevier, Philadelphia, PA, 2010.
[3]     Nicollas R *et al.* "Congenital cysts and fistulas of the neck." *Int J Ped Oto.* 2000; 55: 117-124.
[4]     Pincus RL. "Congenital Neck Masses and Cysts." In: *Head & Neck Surgery – Otolaryngology, 4th Edition.* Bailey BJ *et al.* (Eds.). Lippincott Williams & Wilkins, Philadelphia, PA, 2006.
[5]     Marianowski R *et al.* "Risk factors for thyroglossal duct remnants after Sistrunk procedure in a pediatric population." *Int J Ped Oto* 2003; 67: 19-23.
[6]     Brousseau VJ *et al.* "Thyroglossal duct cysts: presentation and management in children *versus* adults." *Int J Ped Oto.* 2003; 67: 1285-1290.

[7]     Giguere CM *et al.* "New treatment options for lymphangioma in infants and children." *Ann Otol Rhinol Laryngol.* 2002; 111: 1066-1075.

[8]     Maddolozzo JP *et al.* "Congenital Head and Neck Masses." In: *Pediatric Otolaryngology for the Clinician.* Mitchell RB *et al.* (Eds.). Springer, New York, NY, 2009.

[9]     Thorell EA, Chesney PJ. "Cervical Lymphadenitis and Neck Infections." In: *Principles and Practice of Pediatric Diseases Revised, 3rd Edition.* Long SS *et al.* (Eds.). Churchill Livingstone – Elsevier, Philadelphia, PA, 2008.

[10]    Flint D *et al.* "Cervical lymphadenitis due to non-tuberculous mycobacteria: surgical treatment and review." *Int J Ped Oto.* 2000; 53: 187-194.

[11]    O'Handley JG, Tobin EJ, Shah AR. "Otorhinolaryngology." In: *Textbook of Family Medicine, 8th Edition.* Rakel RE and Rakel DP (Eds.). Saunders-Elsevier, Philadelphia, PA, 2011.

[12]    Feder HM and Salazar JC. "A clinical review of 105 patients with PFAPA (a periodic fever syndrome). *Acta Paediatrica.* 2010; 99: 178-184.

[13]    Rogers DA *et al.* "Primary malignancy of the salivary gland in children." *J Ped Surg.* Jan 1994; 29(1): 44-47.

[14]    Zafeiriou DI *et al.* "Congenital Horner's syndrome associated with cervical neuroblastoma." *Eur J Paediatr Neurol* 2006 Mar; 10(2): 90-2.

# CHAPTER 3

## Otitis Media Updates and Current Approaches

## Sven O. Streubel[1] and Hayley L. Ross[2]

*[1]Department of Otolaryngology, Children's Hospital Colorado & University of Colorado School of Medicine, 13123 East 16th Avenue, B455, Aurora, CO 80045, USA and [2]University of Colorado Denver School of Medicine, USA*

**Abstract:** Otitis media (OM) is the most common diagnosis for medical visits in preschool-age children and is the most frequent indication for outpatient antibiotic use in the United States. For any provider who works with pediatric patients, diagnosis and appropriate management of OM is an essential skill, as an estimated 80% of children will suffer from at least one episode in their lifetime. Timely and accurate diagnosis and appropriate management of AOM may have significant consequences for ambulatory health care utilization and expenditures. This chapter addresses the epidemiology, risk factors, pathogenesis, microbiology, diagnosis, treatment and complications of otitis media.

**Keywords:** Otitis media, Acute Otitis Media , Otitis Media with Effusion , Epidemiology, Risk factors, Pathogenesis, Microbiology, Diagnosis, Treatment, Complications, Tympanocentesis, Myringotomy, Otoscopy, Tympanometry, Tympanosclerosis, Cholesteatoma, Tympanic membrane perforation, Hearing loss, Meningitis, Pneumococcal vaccine.

## INTRODUCTION

Otitis media (OM) is the most common diagnosis for medical visits in preschool-age children and is the most frequent indication for outpatient antibiotic use in the United States [1,2]. Management of this diagnosis results in an average expenditure of $350 per child with acute otitis media (AOM), totaling $2.8 billion annually [3]. For any provider who works with pediatric patients, diagnosis and appropriate management of OM is an essential skill, as an estimated 80% of

*Address correspondence to Sven-Orlik Streubel:** The Children's Hospital Otolaryngology, 13123 E. 16th Avenue, B455, Aurora, CO 80045, USA; Tel: (720) 777-8520; Fax: (720) 777-7269; E-mail: Sven.Streubel@childrenscolorado.org

children will suffer from at least one episode in their lifetime [4,5]. Timely and accurate diagnosis and appropriate management of AOM may have significant consequences for ambulatory health care utilization and expenditures.

Otitis media is characterized by signs and symptoms of middle ear effusion, or a fluid collection in the middle ear. It may include otorrhea (drainage of fluid from the middle ear), which occurs after perforation of the tympanic membrane (TM) or through ventilation tubes placed previously. OM is further differentiated by findings on otoscopy.

Despite the widespread incidence, decisions about diagnosis and treatment are complicated. Even the most experienced provider will encounter cases where the diagnosis is not certain. This review is designed to address recent literature on otitis media and serve as a reference for this active area of research.

## DEFINITIONS

Otitis media is divided into two major subclassifications: Acute Otitis Media (AOM) and Otitis Media with Effusion (OME).

AOM is defined by the presence of middle ear inflammation and often presents with constitutional symptoms consistent with infection, such as fever and vomiting.

OME is characterized by middle ear effusion without otalgia, fever and distinct signs of inflammation associated with AOM. Although signs of inflammation are not present, the effusion often becomes colonized with bacteria and may result in AOM.

Treatment-failure AOM is defined as a lack of improvement in signs and symptoms within 48 to 72 hours after initiation of antibiotic therapy.

Recurrent AOM is defined as three or more AOM episodes occurring in the previous 6 months or four or more AOM episodes in the preceding 12 months. OME that persists beyond 3 months is called chronic otitis media or chronic otitis media with effusion.

Chronic suppurative otitis media (CSOM) is defined as purulent otorrhea associated with a chronic tympanic membrane (TM) perforation that persists for more than 6 weeks despite appropriate treatment for AOM.

## EPIDEMIOLOGY AND RISK FACTORS

### Age

The incidence of OM decreases steadily as the age of a child increases. Epidemiologic studies reveal the peak rate of infections occurs in patients between 6 and 18 months [4]. This distribution is likely reflective of increased maturity of the immune system and completion of childhood vaccinations. A decrease in incidence is also observed as the anatomy of the eustachian tube changes with craniofacial maturation, which will be further discussed in another section. The age at first OM diagnosis is inversely related to the relative risk of recurrent episodes [6]. However, the etiology of increased risk is not fully understood.

### Day Care

A number of studies implicate child care outside of the home as a cause for increased rates of AOM. The difference in diagnosis appears to be highest for children prior to age 3 [7,8]. This might be explained by more frequent exposure to pathogens in combination with concombinant limitation in access to breastfeeding, a known protective factor.

### Respiratory Tract Infection

The most commonly identified viral etiologies of OM are rhinovirus and respiratory syncytial virus. However, adenovirus and influenza are often isolated from viral cultures or reverse transcriptase - polymerase chain reaction in up to 43% of patients [9,10]. Viral upper respiratory tract infection (URI) leads to Eustachian tube inflammation resulting in its dysfunction and negative middle ear pressure. This permits secretions containing the infecting virus and pathogenic bacteria that colonize the nasopharynx to enter the middle ear [11]. Animal models have significantly furthered understanding of the contribution of viral infection in the pathogenesis of OM. In the ferret model, infection with influenza A results in ET dysfunction and impairs ventilation of the middle ear. This inability to equalize middle ear pressure contributes to formation of middle ear effusion, which may become superinfected [12]. In the chinchilla, influenza A inoculation significantly increases colonization with *S. pneumoniae* and is correlated with increased rates of OM and a higher proportion of severe infections [13].

## Passive Smoke Exposure

The association between passive smoking and increased childhood URI is well characterized. Chronic exposure results in decreased mucocilliary clearance and induces alteration in mucosal immunity in the respiratory tract. Infants experience AOM and recurrent AOM more frequently than their unexposed counterparts [8]. Interestingly, the available literature suggests that prenatal smoke exposure may increase the risk of disease, while some literature does not show a difference to those only exposed postnatally [14].

## Bottle Feeding or Short Duration of Breast-Feeding

Breast feeding reduces single and recurrent episodes of AOM when breast milk is the only source of nutrition for the first four months of life [8]. Breast milk contains both IgA, which aids in mucosal immunity, and IgG immunoglobulins as well as complement, leukocytes and antioxidants. The protective effect of breast milk is observed even in children with severe craniofacial abnormality. Additionally, the risk for nasopharyngeal aspiration of bottle contents is not insignificant. This can occur particularly when infants are fed by propping a bottle up to the mouth. Tympanometry is a method to measure mobility of the TM and condition of the middle ear. Infants fed by bottle in the horizontal position demonstrated poorer TM function assessed by tympanometry when compared to those fed by breast in the semi-upright position [15].

## Genetics

Twin and sibling studies show an increased risk for OM. This risk is not clearly related to a single gene and is presumed to be multifactorial. Skull, eustachian tube and nasopharyngeal anatomy shared by family members may be the key to the increased incidence. Additionally, variation in immune response to both pathogens and vaccines that target the bacteria of AOM may further alter the frequency of infection. Craniofacial abnormalities such as cleft palate are genetically influenced. Patients with this anatomy are known to have higher incidence and recurrence of OM.

## Nasopharyngeal Colonization

Carriage of *H. influenzae* and *S. pneumoniae* is detectable beginning in infancy. The highest numbers of isolates are found around age 2. In children attending daycare, the spread of nasopharyngeal colonizers is rapid and can include strains of antibiotic resistant *S. pneumoniae*.

## Allergy

Patients who suffer from allergic rhinitis may experience more episodes of OM. There is also evidence that intranasal steroid applied daily may reduce the incidence of recurrent OM. Others found that the diffusion of histamine across the TM leads to altered opening and closing pressures at the tubal orifice, which may explain the mechanism by which infection incidence is increased [16]. Still, the correlation must be better studied to reach consensus. However, the seasonal variation in the diagnosis of OM does not well correlate with the seasonality of allergy. Environmental allergies peak between spring and early fall, while OM occurs most frequently in the winter. Further, atopy in patients with OM was not found to be significantly different. The available evidence is inconclusive at this time and remains controversial.

## PATHOGENESIS

AOM typically occurs after an infection that results in increased congestion of the nasopharynx and eustachian tube. When increased secretions are present, the eustachian tube becomes obstructed and creates persistent negative pressures within the middle ear. Over time, the alteration in pressure can result in reflux of nasopharyngeal contents into the middle ear. Negative pressure also can cause increased vascular permeability and can lead to development of an effusion. In AOM, the effusion contains microorganisms that proliferate in the middle ear and lead to classic symptomatology. Animal models of otitis media are available that successfully replicate middle ear effusion and AOM in the human. Innoculation of rat model ears with *S. pneumoniae* and *M. catarrhalis* showed that the presence of bacteria can induce cytokine expression [17]. Many of the activated cytokines are potent inducers of TNF-alpha, which in turn recruits neutrophils and mediates much of the destructive process in the middle ear. Work in the chinchilla led to the discovery of biofilm production by H. influenzae, which aids in bacterial evasion of the host defenses.

## EUSTACHIAN TUBE ANATOMY

The anatomy of the eustachian tube (ET) and middle ear also impacts the propensity toward infection. Imaging of the temporal bone demonstrates that the average volume of the middle ear is approximately 1.5 times larger in the adult than in the infant. Similarly, the ET lumen is larger in the adult ear [18,19]. Further the ossified proportion of the ET increases as the patient ages and the angle of entry into the middle ear becomes more lateral with time. Maturation of the paratubal muscles occurs with aging. All of these factors contribute to more efficient opening, ventilation and mucocilliary clearance. Studies of patients born with craniofacial abnormalities add further evidence to the role of ET maturation in the pathogenesis of OM. Histologic studies of ET tissue from children born with cleft lip or palate shows evidence of immaturity of the cartilaginous tissue of the tube, which may partially explain the higher propensity toward infection in those children. Similarly, imaging studies demonstrate a more horizontal orientation of the tube, allowing for more direct entry of bacteria into the middle ear. Eustachian tube manometry is used to better characterize the function of the tube. However, clinical studies do not show clear prognostic value in routine manometry and it is currently used primarily in the research setting.

## MICROBIOLOGY

Viral infection, particularly upper respiratory infection is felt to be the common antecedent event in the development of OM. Cultured viruses are often Respiratory Syncytial Virus (RSV), Parainfluenza or Influenza viruses. The mechanism of this predisposing infection for development of OM is multifactorial. Viral upper respiratory infections can lead to bacterial superinfection and induce the production of cytokines. The cascade results in the final production of TNF-alpha, which appears to mediate much of the inflammatory processes in AOM. There also appears to be a synergistic effect of some bacteria that cause AOM with viral infections. In cultures of middle ear fluid, coinfection with influenza virus results in increased colonization of *S. pneumoniae* in the middle ear [13]. Viral infection may also facilitate adherence of bacteria by exposing receptors previously unavailable to the bacteria. The overall incidence of URI complicated by otitis media has been reported to be 61% in children between 6 months and 3 years of age, with a 37% incidence of AOM and 24% incidence of OME [20]. Tympanocentesis is a reliable method for pathogen identification. Swabs from the nasopharynx or throat are insensitive and specimens are often contaminated with normal flora. Viruses are the most common cause of OM, but traditional viral cultures are often negative when tympanocentesis is performed. The use of DNA and RNA probes as well as antigen tests have increased the sensitivity of culture. For the routine patient, cultures are unnecessary. Still, there is data to support the use of antiviral medications in the prevention of OM. Administration of oseltamivir to children with influenza has shown to reduce episodes of OM by 44% [21]. This is not routinely done in clinical practice and may necessitate confirmation of virus type prior to use of an antiviral. Multiple studies have shown a modest reduction in the incidence of culture-positive influenza AOM. However, the benefit is much stronger in patients receiving a live attenuated vaccine as opposed to the more commonly administered trivalent inactivated immunization [22,23]. The three most common cultured bacteria responsible for infection are *S. pneumoniae, H. influenzae,* and *M. catarrhalis.* Historically, the role of *S. pneumoniae* is well established; it was first described as the cause of otitis media in 1888 [4]. These bacteria are not routine colonizers in the EAC, but are frequently found in the nasopharynx, which further supports the mechanism of infection from nasopharyngeal region as previously described [24]. The majority of infections are caused by *S. pneumoniae* or *H. influenzae,* and there is regional variation in the most common pathogen. Clinical evidence indicates that *S. pneumoniae* is a more virulent pathogen in the middle ear and is more often recovered from recurrent cases of AOM or after treatment failures. Some studies have found that *S. pneumoniae* infection can lead to a higher fever and more toxic appearance of the patient [25]. However, there is no known otoscopic difference between those pathogens. The advent of the pneumococcal conjugate vaccine provides protection against some of the S. pneumoniae serotypes implicated in AOM. While not beneficial in the acute treatment, several studies have shown decreased office visits and diagnosis of otitis in patients who complete the three shot primary pneumococcal conjugate series (PCV) [26,27].

*H. influenzae* is frequently isolated from the nasopharynx and may be carried by up to half of all children [28]. Prior to the availability of the *H. influenzae* type b vaccine series, approximately 10% of cases were due to typable Haemophilus b strains. Though this species is not the primary pathogen in most childhood cases, it is a commonly isolated cause of OM in older children and adults [29].

Moraxella species are also common colonizers of the nasopharynx in children and infants. Interestingly, cases of OM in which *M. catarrhalis* was isolated were rare until the 1980s but have increased in frequency in recent years.

*Group A Streptococci, Staphylococcus aureus* and gram-negative bacilli are responsible for the minority of infections. Isolation of *S. aureus* or *P. aeruginosa* in particular may indicate underlying systemic disease such as HIV or diabetes. Group A species, more often found in cases of pharyngitis, may cause OM through direct alteration of eustachian tube function. However, it is not currently a significant pathogen.

**DIAGNOSIS**

Accurate diagnosis of OM presents a challenge, particularly for children under 2 years of age. Appropriate use of diagnostic criteria is essential to prevent complications, while minimizing overuse of antibiotics. The history and overall clinical picture is useful in determining which children may benefit from treatment.

The diagnosis of AOM is based in large part on history and behavior of the child. In 2004, the American Academy of Pediatrics and the American Academy of Family Practice published new Clinical Practice Guidelines on Acute Otitis Media, clarifying diagnostic criteria. Patients typically contract an initial URI and later develop otalgia, fever, and systemic symptoms such as irritability, anorexia, and vomiting. Otoscopy may reveal loss of bony landmarks, bulging or poor mobility of the TM.

Otitis media with effusion may present long after the effusion develops, as children are often minimally symptomatic. Patients commonly complain of hearing loss and may describe tinnitus or vertigo. Older children describe feelings of aural fullness. Otoscopic findings are often similar to that of AOM. The overlap on physical exam of the patient may make differentiation between AOM and OME difficult. This is particularly true if findings are noted on routine exam and the patient has not developed fever or otalgia. Even the use of the diagnostic aids below may leave the diagnosis uncertain, as most are not sensitive for AOM. In these cases, it may be useful to provide parents with careful return precautions and consider supplying reliable families with a prescription to be filled if symptoms worsen.

## Blood Culture

Bacteriemia in otitis media is rare. In a study by Teele *et al.* blood cultures were drawn from all patients presenting to an ambulatory setting with fever. Of the 166 patients subsequently diagnosed with otitis, only 1.2% were bacteremic [30]. The sensitivity for diagnosis and identification of a pathogen is extremely low, but may be useful in particularly ill children who have complications of otitis media such as meningitis.

## Leukocyte Count, C-Reactive Protein, and Erythrocyte Sedimentation Rate

Routine serum testing is typically unnecessary in uncomplicated cases of otitis media. However, there is evidence to suggest that the mean leukocyte count may be higher in patients with AOM than counterparts with effusion alone. Similarly, the sedimentation rate is higher in patients with bacterial pathogens in the middle ear effusion. No difference has been show in C-reactive protein levels regardless of presence of bacteria in the middle ear.

## Otoscopy and Pneumatic Otoscopy

Clearance of cerumen from the external auditory canal is essential to proper examination of the tympanic membrane (TM). Visualization of the TM is required to make an accurate diagnosis. If otoscopic microscopes are available, a curette may be used to gently clean the canal. Suction with a fine tip is also helpful. Lavage of the canal is generally appropriate for older children who can cooperate with the examiner and remain still.

Current literature indicates that pneumatic otoscopy is the most accurate method of diagnosis when used by an experienced clinician. However, routine use in clinical practice is variable and the accuracy of the diagnosis may be dependent on the comfort of the examiner [31,32]. Training and routine use of this technique is essential to increasing diagnostic utility. Common barriers to correct use include a poor seal between the speculum and the canal, which renders the technique ineffective. Therefore, it is important to select the largest possible speculum that is tolerable for the child.

It is important to note that the sensitivity and specificity of this technique applies only to pneumatic otoscopy, not otoscopy alone. Commonly used diagnostic criteria such as erythema of the TM may be nonspecific signs of fever or crying.

## Tympanometry

This technique is used frequently on children of young age or those who require ear surgery. However, it is relatively simple to perform on a routine basis and may be more effective in the diagnosis for infants. This technique measures compliance of the TM and can provide information on the presence of effusion, Eustachian tube function and normality of the TM. This technique is accurate for diagnosis of middle ear effusion and is relatively simple to perform with proper training. However, there is no information provided about the presence or absence of inflammation in the middle ear. Therefore, use of tympanometry cannot be applied to diagnose AOM, but may provide additional information should signs and symptoms of inflammation be present and is reliable in the diagnosis of OME. Highly negative pressures are typically abnormal, but may vary with season, concomitant respiratory infection or be a physiologic variant.

## Tympanocentesis

Tympanocentesis confirms the presence of an effusion. Aspiration of fluid provides a sample for culture so that targeted therapy may be used. Still, tympanocentesis is not performed for routine AOM as empiric treatment or observation often result in improvement of symptoms. The procedure is indicated for treatment failure after two complete courses of empiric antibiotics, sepsis evaluation, mastoiditis, or for patients with immune deficiency. It is also performed in the research setting. Culture data from tympanocentesis provided valuable information on the microbiology of middle ear infection.

## Acoustic Reflexometry

This method measures changes in the TM that can be correlated with measurement of middle ear pressure and is useful in diagnosing effusion. The advantage of this technique is that a tight seal is not necessary for proper use. Acoustic reflexometry is not currently available in routine clinical use [33].

## TREATMENT

While the diagnosis of AOM can be complicated, the judicious use of antibiotics in this illness is difficult. Providers must weigh carefully the goal of improved symptoms and prevention of potential complications against over prescribing antibiotics. In strains of *S. pneumoniae*, a number of resistant strains are colonizers in the nasopharynx that circulate in the community. Additionally, development of novel resistant strains is quite rapid [34].

### The Role of Observation

In efforts to reduce overuse of antibiotics and minimize unnecessary side effects, careful observation is warranted. By 24 hours after diagnosis, 61% of children who have AOM have decreased symptoms, whether they receive placebo or antibiotics, and by 1 week, approximately 75% have resolution of their symptoms [35]. The AAP/AFP Guidelines released in 2004 suggest observation in a selected group of patients. This option may be considered in non-toxic appearing patients who are older than age 2. Younger children or those who demonstrate severe otalgia, bilateral infection, high or persistent fever should not be managed with observation, but should be treated with antibiotics [36].

### Antibiotic Therapy

Many isolates of *S. pneumoniae* circulating in the community have some level of antibiotic resistance. However, Amoxicillin remains an effective treatment option. Much of the effect of antibiotic resistance can be overcome by providing high dosages to the child, which carries little additional risk. Oral cephalosporins such as cefdinir and cefuroxime are effective options for children with sensitivity to Amoxicillin. When studied with amoxicillin-clavulanate in a double-blinded RCT, rates of treatment failure are equal. However, amoxicillin-clavulanate carries the added benefit of potential eradication of colonizing *S. pneumoniae* flora [37]. Overall, these medications may be more difficult to use for a complete course, as their taste is less acceptable to patients than amoxicillin. For patients experiencing severe pain and temperature greater than 39.0°C, high-dose amoxicillin-clavulanate (90 mg/kg per day amoxicillin; 6.4 mg/kg per day clavulanate) is recommended as initial therapy. For treatment of clinical failure 3 days into antibiotic therapy, the AAP suggests high-dose amoxicillin-clavulanate (90 mg/kg per day amoxicillin; 6.4 mg/kg per day clavulanate) or intramuscular ceftriaxone for 1 to 3 days.

For patients with a type I penicillin allergy the AAP recommends the use of azalides or macrolides such as azithromycin (10 mg/kg per day on day 1 followed by 5 mg/kg per day for 4 days as a single daily dose) and clarithromycin (15 mg/kg per day in two divided doses for 10 days or for 5 to 7 days if > 6 years of age and has mild-to-moderate disease). However, a substantial proportion of *S pneumoniae* organisms are resistant to these agents. Patients who have severe disease should receive a combination of clindamycin (30 to 40 mg/kg per day in three divided doses) to cover *S. pneumoniae* and sulfisoxazole for nontypeable *H influenzae*. Those patients who have nontype I penicillin allergies should be prescribed oral cephalosporins such as cefdinir (14 mg/kg per day divided twice a day or daily, with twice-daily therapy approved for 5 to 10 days), cefuroxime (30 mg/kg per day in two divided doses), cefpodoxime (10 mg/kg per day once daily), or intramuscular ceftriaxone (50 mg/kg for 1 to 3 days) [36]. Overall, longer therapy duration is shown to be more effective at treating acute infection, but does not show long term benefit in preventing relapse [38]. Tympanocentesis helps guide therapy in patients who are severely ill and have failed second-line antibiotic management or in those who have failed first-line agents and who also have a penicillin allergy. Tympanocentesis should also be strongly considered for immunocompromised patients, neonates younger than 2 weeks of age, and patients who have AOM that has been refractory to treatment or if AOM is present in infants within the first 2 months of birth to identify the causative organisms and target antibiotic therapy more accurately. For patients who require alternate antibiotic therapy, fluoroquniolones are appropriate options. Many isolates of *S. pneumoniae* are susceptible to the quinolones. They are not routinely used in the pediatric population as they are not well studied in patients less than 16 and carry a proportionally higher rate of adverse side effects. Trimethoprim-sulfamethoxasole has also been studied, which demonstrated high rates of eradication, but rapid development of resistance [39].

## Ventilation

Myringotomy and pressure equalization tube placement (PET) is a standard surgical treatment of acute otitis media and recurrent OME. The benefit of PET placement is realized in the reduction of illnesses and preservation of hearing. Although there is no rigid guideline for tube placement, the clinician should consider the developmental stage of the child and the frequency of illness each year. If the patient is at a time of rapid language acquisition, PET placement may minimize potential speech and hearing delays. As fluid is drained from the middle ear, the conductive hearing loss associated is minimized. However, the potential for tympanosclerosis, discussed below, which can also cause long term conductive damage remains after tympanostomy tubes are placed.

## Prevention

One of the greatest impacts on incidence and microbiology of AOM is the advent of routine vaccination. In a study by Eskola *et al.* the multivalent pneumococcal vaccine (PCV7) reduced the number of episodes of AOM due to any cause by 6%, reduced culture-confirmed pneumococcal AOM episodes by 34%, and reduced the number of AOM episodes due to serotypes contained in PCV7 by 57% [27]. The number of episodes caused by cross-reactive serotypes decreased by 51%; the number of episodes due to all other serotypes actually increased by 33%. A Kaiser Permanente study involving 37,868 children who were randomized to receive PCV7 or placebo found that children who received the primary series of PCV7 had a reduction of otitis media visits by 7.8%, of antibiotic prescriptions by 5.7%, and of tympanostomy tube placements by 24% [26]. For recurrent AOM, PCV7 reduced the risk of three visits by 10% and the risk of 10 visits by 20% within a 6-month period. In addition, Poehling and associates reported a 17% to 28% reduction in the frequency of AOM and a 16% to 23% reduction in the frequency of tympanostomy tube placements from pre-PCV7 to post-PCV7 [40]. Unfortunately serotypes included in the vaccine are replaced by other serotypes not susceptible to Penicillin and other antibiotics causing local and invasive pneumococcal disease. The Centers for Disease Control and Prevention have documented that the annual incidence of pneumococcal disease due to nonvaccine serotypes in children younger than 5 years of age has increased from an average of 16.3 cases per 100,000 population during prevaccine years (1998 to 1999) to 19.9 cases per 100,000 population in 2004.

A number of other preventive measures are proposed. Use of intranasal antibiotics shows some promise for reducing recurrent cases in patients with frequent AOM. Use of Xylitol gum has also been studied, but is shown to be useful only in a small age range of children with consistent use [41]. Tonsillectomy with or without adenoidectomy has been proposed. Given the necessity of proper ET function, the surgery makes intuitive sense, though showed only very modest benefit in a recent randomized trial and no effect for adenoidectomy alone [42].

Antibiotic prophylaxis with amoxicillin is not routinely recommended as more frequent use contributes to increased antibiotic resistance. However, studies show that prophylaxis does reduce the incidence of OM in patients prone to infection.

Finally, education of caregivers and minimizing risk factors in the home environment is beneficial. Although many factors that are known to increase risk of OM are not modifiable, parents may be motivated to reduce cigarette smoke exposure or minimize time in day care if possible.

## COMPLICATIONS

Apart from the acute symptoms, sequelae of otitis media can lead to complications into adulthood. These events range from significant intracranial complications to speech delay.

### Tympanic Membrane

*Tympanosclerosis*

The presence of a white and calcified appearance of the TM is the common finding of myringosclerosis or tympanosclerosis. Myringosclerosis involves the

TM alone, while tympanosclerosis affects the tympanum, or middle ear. This process is the final result of inflammation or trauma to the ear, including placement of ventilation tubes. These plaques are comprised of hyaline cartilage and are followed by accumulation of calcium and phosphate crystals. The pathogenesis is not fully understood, but cytokines appear to play a role in the activation of osteoclast-like cells [43]. Studies have demonstrated a male predominance in the development of tympanosclerosis [44]. With time, tympanosclerosis can lead to hearing loss, as tympanic membrane mobility changes. Plaques may also accumulate on the ossicles and limit mobility of the bones.

### Tympanic Membrane Perforation

Perforation is a common complication of AOM. Patients often present with otorrhea and may experience an improvement in otalgia after perforation occurs. These perforations can often be managed conservatively and may heal spontaneously by migration of epithelium over the defect. Perforations that do not heal after 3 months are unlikely to heal spontaneously, even though complete resolution of AOM occurs [31]. Referral to an otolaryngologist is indicated in these patients.

### Cholesteatoma

A pearly appearance within the middle ear or mastoid is often indicative of cholesteatoma. This benign cyst is actually filled primarily with keratin and epithelial debris, not cholesterol. Cholesteatomas occur congenitally as well, but are also sequelae of otitis media or trauma. The pathogenesis is not fully understood, but may involve migration of epithelial tissue through a preexisting defect. Metaplasia of middle ear cells has also been proposed. Although these collections of debris are not malignant, they enlarge with time and may result in fistula formation, hearing loss due to ossicular chain damage, and can become colonized with bacteria and infected.

### Atelectasis

Atelectasis is a retraction of a portion or the entirety of the TM. Development occurs when pressures in the middle ear cannot be appropriately equalized, which is the result of eustachian tube dysfunction. When this fails to occur normally, as in frequent episodes of AOM, the TM can become retracted onto the ossicles. Retraction onto the bones of the middle ear can lead to decreased mobility of the eardrum and ultimately to hearing loss.

## Persistent Middle Ear Effusion

The presence of middle ear effusion following an episode of AOM may be referred to as persistent MEE. The effusion can remain for multiple weeks or months after the resolution of AOM.

## Facial Paralysis

The facial nerve passes through the middle ear as it travels to innervate the muscles of facial expression. Paralysis can be acutely observed as inflammation and infection impacts nerve function and may be associated with mastoiditis, with osteitis or abscess. Many patients will have full restoration of their facial strength. In fact, most patients can be successfully treated by administration of appropriate antibiotics, myringotomy with or without tube placement and tympanocentesis [45].

## Hearing Loss

The mechanism of hearing loss in patients after otitis media occurs through direct destruction of the middle ear structures (ossicular damage, tympanosclerosis or TM abnormalities), OME or persistent MEE, and/or chronic auditory deprivation. Hearing loss can be primarily sensorineural, conductive or mixed. Patients who develop acute loss of hearing due to middle ear effusion typically return to their baseline level of function. Those who develop sensorineural loss are less likely to recover, as this most often represents extension of infection into the structures of the inner ear. Regardless of the primary mechanism, complications of OM are among the leading cause of acquired hearing loss.

In a study of children ages 3 through 6 years, hearing loss was documented after the diagnosis of AOM or OME. Deficits averaged about 20 dB in affected children and a policy of watchful waiting was implemented [46]. Many children recovered to their pre-illness baseline without any intervention. Again, though many children recover well from AOM or OME, there isn't currently enough literature available to suggest which children may go on to recover spontaneously and which will require intervention from an otolaryngologist in the future. The available evidence supports referral if effusion persists for over three months [31].

## Speech and Development

Frequent AOM and OME impacts the development of a child in more than simply missed time from school and other educational opportunities. In recent years, a number of studies have characterized the impact of frequent AOM, chronic otitis media or otitis with effusion on speech and development. Mody *et al.* found that children with a history of OME during the first year of life had difficulty with speech perception compared to peers with no history [47]. The prevalence of OME by age 2 years also appears to impact discrimination of sound in older children, with a difference noted in those older than 7 years.

The available literature supports a difference in speech perception, but randomized controlled studies have not found a relationship between frequency of AOM or OME and articulation or new word acquisition. Further, children undergoing immediate ventilation tube surgery do not score better than peers who received tube placement after a longer observation period.

## Mastoiditis

Mastoiditis is inflammation of the mastoid process and air cell system. The infection occurs by direct extension from the middle ear into the air cells or by venous drainage in the mastoid. Mastoiditis is a spectrum of disease, which includes isolated infection of the air cells, infection of the periosteum or osteum. Subacute and chronic processes also occur. Patients with infection of the air cells without further involvement will often experience spontaneous resolution, but may go on to develop further spread of infection.

Notably, this complication can occur with a child's first episode of AOM. In fact, most children do not have any history of recurrent ear infection and mastoiditis may be the first sign of any ear pathology. Acute mastoiditis with periostitis or osteitis should be suspected whenever projection of the pinnae is observed.

Tenderness, swelling over the mastoid process, otorrhea, post auricular pain and fever are also common hallmarks. The presence of an abscess in the neck, or Bezold abscess, may be observed. CT or MRI are both appropriate imaging modalities to characterize the extent of disease.

As the primary pathogenesis is through direct extension of the infection into the mastoid system, the common pathogens are similar to the frequently observed agents in AOM. Additionally, S. aureus and Pseudomonas aeruginosa are commonly isolated. With the availability of antibiotics, surgical intervention is not always necessary. However, after several years of stability, the incidence of mastoiditis is on the rise. Many hypothesize that this is representative of increasing rates of resistance and changing patterns of infectious agents. The majority of cases can still be managed with intravenous antibiotics. A recent study found only 23.8% of patients treated with early antibiotics required cortical mastoidectomy and myringotomy [48].

**Intracranial Complications**

Despite the widespread use of antibiotics intracranial complications occur with relatively high frequency. Meningitis is most common and results from direct extension of infection through the dura. Brain abscess, epidural abscess and sinus thrombosis occur rarely. Babin *et al.* [40] reported that the presenting symptoms of meningitis include otorrhea, fever, and otalgia. The presence of neurologic symptoms should raise concern with the relatively nonspecific otologic complaints. Some authors have found that a severe earache or localized pain over the affected ear may occur in addition to vertigo, headache, and meningeal signs. Abscesses can often be identified with a contrast CT of the temporal bones. Imaging also helps to characterize the degree of involvement of the mastoid.

Although intracranial involvement is a less common complication, the mortality of and morbidity is high. Babin *et al.* found that 26% of patients died after an intracranial process was diagnosed and a significant proportion of survivors had long term morbidity [49]. Patients who experience coma as result of their illness and those with elevated erythrocyte sedimentation rates have the worst prognosis. However, prompt administration of appropriate antibiotics and the involvement of our neurosurgery colleagues may improve the prognosis of this devastating complication.

## Chronic Otitis Media

As previously described, COM or *chronic suppurative otitis media* is persistent otorrhea after PET placement or through a perforated TM. This sequela may occur through similar pathogenesis as the acute infection, or result from deposition of external ear flora through the perforated or intubated TM. The microbiology of COM initially contains isolates from *S. pneumonia* and *H. influenzae* when otorrhea first develops. Over time the primary pathogens become *Pseudomonas aeruginosa* and *Staphylococcus aureus*.

Treatment of COM requires appropriate coverage of organisms and can be administered through otic drops or oral therapy. Meticulous aural hygiene is essential with the goal of maintaining a dry ear. These patients are at risk for intracranial complications and should be managed in consultation with an otolaryngologist.

## Petrositis

Petrositis is the result of direct extension of infection from the middle ear and mastoid to the petrous portion of the temporal bone. Gradenigo's triad, which includes classical symptoms of otitis media, deep facial pain and ipsilateral paralysis of the abducens nerve is rare. However, deep facial pain and the presence of otorrhea should raise suspicion for petrositis. As with mastoiditis, systemic antibiotic therapy may be able to adequately address the infection [50]. If surgical therapy is required, drainage of the apical portion of the petrous bone is attempted through the middle ear and mastoid.

## Sigmoid Sinus Thrombosis

In the era of antibiotics, sigmoid sinus thrombosis also became a rare complication. The morbidity and mortality have fallen with routine use of antibiotics and mastoidectomy. Diagnosis is best made with MRI imagining of the cerebral vasculature. Administration of antibiotics and mastoidectomy are the preferred method of treatment. Anticoagulation is a safe alternative if surgical options are not available [51].

## Otic Hydrocephalus

Although a rare complication of OM, otic hydrocephalus can range in severity from mild headache to progression to coma and death. The pathogenesis is not fully understood, it likely results from reduced venous flow and occlusion of the lateral or sigmoid sinus [52]. Therefore it is a heterogeneous condition in which an otic cause is attributed to symptoms and findings of acute hydrocephalus. If suspected, emergent CT scan should be performed and the patient should be managed in consult with neurosurgery.

## REFERRAL TO AN OTOLARYNGOLOGIST

The majority of cases of otitis media are well within the scope of management by the primary care provider. Providers who care for children may consider referral of any patient who experiences hearing loss, perforation, or persistent otorrhea. Medical management can suffice for these conditions, but surgery options are often available and indicated.

## ACKNOWLEDGEMENT

Declared none.

## CONFLICT OF INTEREST

The authors confirm that this chapter content has no conflict of interest.

## REFERENCES

[1]     Schappert S. Office visits for otitis media: United States, 1975–1990. *Adv Data Vital Health Stat.* 1992;214:1–20.

[2]     McCaig LF HJ. Trends in antimicrobial drug prescribing among office-based physicians in the United States. *JAMA: the journal of the American Medical Association.* 1995; 273(3):214-219.

[3]     Soni A. Ear Infections (Otitis Media) in Children (0–17): Use and Expenditures, 2006. *Statistical Brief No. 228. Agency for Healthcare Research and Quality.* \. 2008. Available at: http://www.meps.ahrq.gov/mepsweb     /data_files/publications/st228/stat228.pdf. Accessed September 20, 2010.

[4]     Bluestone CD, Klein JO. Otitis Media and Eustachian Tube Dysfunction. In: Bluestone CD, Stool SE, Alper CM, *et al.*, eds. *Pediatric Otolaryngology.* 4th ed. Philadelphia: Saunders; 2003:488-547.

[5]     Gates G. Acute otitis media and otitis media with effusion. In: Cummings C, ed. *Otolaryngology- Head and Neck Surgery*. 3rd ed. St. Louis: Mosby; 1998.

[6]     Teele DW, Klein JO, Bratton L, Fisch GR, Mathieu OR, Porter PJ, Starobin SG, Tarlin LD YR. Use of pneumococcal vaccine for prevention of recurrent acute otitis media in infants in Boston. The Greater Boston Collaborative Otitis Media Study Group. *Rev Infect Dis*. 1981;3(Suppl):S113-8.

[7]     Network NI of CH and HDECCR. Child care and common communicable illnesses in children aged 37 to 54 months. *Archives of pediatrics & adolescent medicine*. 2003;157(2):196-200.

[8]     Uhari M, Mantysaari K, Niemela M. REVIEW ARTICLE A Meta-Analytic Review of the Risk Factors for Acute Otitis Media. *Clinical Infectious Diseases*. 1996;(January):1079-1083.

[9]     Ishibashi T, Monobe H, Nomura Y, Shinogami M YJ. Multiplex nested reverse transcription-polymerase chain reaction for respiratory viruses in acute otitis media. *Annals of Otology, Rhinology & Laryngology*. 2003;112(3):252-7.

[10]    Vesa S, Kleemola M, Blomqvist S, *et al*. Epidemiology of documented viral respiratory infections and acute otitis media in a cohort of children followed from two to twenty-four months of age. *The Pediatric infectious disease journal*. 2001;20(6):574-81.

[11]    Bakaletz L. Viral potentiation of bacterial superinfection of the respiratory tract. *Trends in Microbiology*. 1995;3(3):110-114.

[12]    Buchman C a, Swarts JD, Seroky JT, *et al*. Otologic and systemic manifestations of experimental influenza A virus infection in the ferret. *Otolaryngology--head and neck surgery*. 1995;112(4):572-8.

[13]    Tong H, Fisher L, Kosunick G, DeMaria T. Effect of adenovirus type 1 and influenza A virus on Streptococcus pneumoniae nasopharyngeal colonization and otitis media in the chinchilla. *Annals of Otology, Rhinology & Laryngology*. 2000;109(11):1021-7.

[14]    Stathis S, O'Callaghan D, Williams G, *et al*. Maternal cigarette smoking during pregnancy is an independent predictor for symptoms of middle ear disease at five years' postdelivery. *Pediatrics*. 1999;104:e16.

[15]    Tully S, Bar-Haim Y, Bradley R. Abnormal tympanography after supine bottle feeding. *Journal of Pediatrics*. 1995;126:S:105.

[16]    Friedman R, Doyle W, Casselbrant M, Bluestone C, Fireman P. Immunologic-mediated eustachian tube obstruction: a double-blind crossover study. *Journal of Allergy and Clinical Immunology*. 1981;71(5):442-7.

[17]    Melhus A, Ryan A. Expression of cytokine genes during pneumococcal and nontypeable Haemophiius influenzae acute otitis media in the rat. *Infect Immun*. 2000;68(7):4024-31.

[18]    Ishijima K, Sando I, Miura M, Balaban CD, Takasaki K SM. Postnatal development of static volume of the eustachian tube lumen. A computer-aided three-dimensional reconstruction and measurement study. *Annals of Otology, Rhinology & Laryngology*. 2002;111(9):832-5.

[19]    Ikui A, Sando I, Haginomori S-ichi, *et al*. Postnatal Development of the Tympanic Cavity a Computer-aided reconstruction and measurement study. *Acta Otolaryngology*. 2000;120(3):375-379.

[20]    Chonmaitree T, Revai K, Grady JJ, *et al*. Viral upper respiratory tract infection and otitis media complication in young children. *Clinical infectious diseases: an official publication of the Infectious Diseases Society of America*. 2008;46(6):815-23.

[21]    Whitley R, Hayden E, Reisinger K. Oral oseltamivir treatment of influenza in children. *Pediatr Infect Dis J.* 2001;20(2):127-33.

[22]    Block SL, Heikkinen T, Toback SL, Zheng W, Ambrose CS. The efficacy of live attenuated influenza vaccine against influenza-associated acute otitis media in children. *The Pediatric infectious disease journal.* 2011;30(3):203-7.

[23]    Belshe RB, Edwards KM, Vesikari T, *et al.* Live attenuated *versus* inactivated influenza vaccine in infants and young children. *The New England journal of medicine.* 2007;356(7):685-96.

[24]    Stenfors L-E, Raisanen S. Quantity of aerobic bacteria in the bony portion of the external auditory canal of children. *International Journal of Pediatric Otorhinolaryngology.* 2002;66(2):167-173.

[25]    Rodriguez W, Schwartz R. Streptococcus pneumoniae causes otitis media with higher fever and more redness of tympanic membranes than Haemophilus influenzae or Moraxella catarrhalis. *Pediatric Infectious Disease Journal.* 1999;18(10):942.

[26]    Fireman B, Black SB, Shinefield HR, *et al.* Impact of the pneumococcal conjugate vaccine on otitis media. *The Pediatric infectious disease journal.* 2003;22(1):10-6.

[27]    Eskola J, Kilpi T, Palmu A, *et al.* Efficacy of a Pneumococcal Conjugate Vaccine against Acute Otitis Media. *New England Journal of Medicine.* 2001;344(6):403-409.

[28]    Faden H, Duffy L, Wasielewski R, *et al.* Relationship between nasopharyngeal colonization and the development of otitis media in children. Tonawanda/Williamsville Pediatrics. *The Journal of infectious diseases.* 1997;175(6):1440-5.

[29]    Schwartz R, Rodriguez W. Acute otitis media in children eight years old and older: a reappraisal of the role of Hemophilus influenzae. *American Journal of Otolaryngology.* 1981;2(1):19-21.

[30]    Teele D, Pelton S, Grant M. Bacteremia in febrile children under 2 years of age: results of cultures of blood of 600 consecutive febrile children seen in a walk-in clinic. *Journal of Pediatrics1.* 1975;87(2):227-230.

[31]    Rosenfeld RM, Culpepper L, Doyle KJ, *et al.* Clinical practice guideline: Otitis media with effusion. *Otolaryngology--head and neck surgery: official journal of American Academy of Otolaryngology-Head and Neck Surgery.* 2004;130(5 Suppl):S95-118.

[32]    Steinbach W, Sectish T, Benjamin DJ, Chang K, Messner A. Pediatric residents' clinical diagnostic accuracy of otitis media. *Pediatrics.* 2002;109(6):993-8.

[33]    Kemaloğlu YK, Beder L, Sener T, Göksu N. Tympanometry and acoustic reflectometry in ears with chronic retraction without effusion. *International journal of pediatric otorhinolaryngology.* 2000;55(1):21-7.

[34]    Dagan R, Leibovitz E, Cheletz G, Leiberman A, Porat N. Antibiotic treatment in acute Otitis Media promotes superinfection with resistant Streptococcus pneumoniae carried before initiation of treatment. *The Journal of infectious diseases.* 2001;183(6):880-6.

[35]    Rosenfeld R, Kay D. Natural history of untreated otitis media. In: Rosenfeld R, Bluestone C, eds. *Evidence-based Otitis Media.* 2nd ed. Ontario: Hamilton; 2003:180–198.

[36]    Practice AA of P and AA of F. Diagnosis and Management of Acute Otitis Media. *Pediatrics.* 2004;113(5):1451-1465.

[37]    Block SL, McCarty JM, Hedrick J a, *et al.* Comparative safety and efficacy of cefdinir *vs.* amoxicillin/clavulanate for treatment of suppurative acute otitis media in children. *The Pediatric infectious disease journal.* 2000;19(12 Suppl):S159-65.

[38]   Cohen R, Levy C, Boucherat M, *et al.* Five *vs.* ten days of antibiotic therapy for acute otitis media in young children. *The Pediatric infectious disease journal.* 2000;19(5):458-63. Available at: http://www.ncbi.nlm.nih.gov/pubmed/10819344.

[39]   Leiberman A, Leibovitz E, Piglansky L, *et al.* Bacteriologic and clinical efficacy of trimethoprim-sulfamethoxazole for treatment of acute otitis media. *The Pediatric infectious disease journal.* 2001;20(3):260-4.

[40]   Poehling K a, Lafleur BJ, Szilagyi PG, *et al.* Population-based impact of pneumococcal conjugate vaccine in young children. *Pediatrics.* 2004;114(3):755-61.

[41]   Tapiainen T, Luotonen L, Kontiokari T, Renko M, Uhari M. Xylitol administered only during respiratory infections failed to prevent acute otitis media. *Pediatrics.* 2002;109(2):E19.

[42]   Oomen KPQ, Rovers MM, van den Akker EH, *et al.* Effect of adenotonsillectomy on middle ear status in children. *The Laryngoscope.* 2005;115(4):731-4.

[43]   Makiishi-Shimobayashi C, Tsujimura T, Sugihara A, *et al.* Expression of osteopontin by exudate macrophages in inflammatory tissues of the middle ear: a possible association with development of tympanosclerosis. *Hearing research.* 2001;153(1-2):100-7.

[44]   Koc A, Uneri C. Sex distribution in children with tympanosclerosis after insertion of a tympanostomy tube. *European archives of oto-rhino-laryngology : official journal of the European Federation of Oto-Rhino-Laryngological Societies (EUFOS) : affiliated with the German Society for Oto-Rhino-Laryngology - Head and Neck Surgery.* 2001;258(1):16-9.

[45]   Bluestone C, Klein J. Intratemporal Complications and Sequelae of Otitis Media Bluestone CD, Stool SE, Alper CM, *et al.*, eds. *Pediatric Otolaryngology.* 2003:687-763.

[46]   Fria T, EI C, Eichler J. Hearing acuity of children with otitis media with effusion. *Arch Otolaryngology.* 1985;111(1):10-16.

[47]   Mody M, Schwartz R, Gravel J, Ruben R. Speech perception and verbal memory in children with and without histories of otitis media. *Journal of speech, language and hearing research.* 1999;42(5):1069-79.

[48]   De S, Makura ZGG, Clarke RW. Paediatric acute mastoiditis: the Alder Hey experience. *The Journal of laryngology and otology.* 2002;116(6):440-2.

[49]   Babin E, Brenac F, Bequignon A. Intracranial complications of acute mastoiditis. *Ann Otolaryngol Chir Cervicofac.* 2001;118(5):323-9.

[50]   Burston BJ, Pretorius PM, Ramsden JD. Gradenigo ' s syndrome : successful conservative treatment in adult and paediatric patients. *The Journal of Laryngology & Otology.* 2005;119(April):325-329.

[51]   Ropposch T, Nemetz U, Braun E, *et al.* Management of otogenic sigmoid sinus thrombosis. *Otology & Neurotology.* 2011;32(7):1120-3.

[52]   El-Kashlan HK, Harker LA, Shelton C, Aygun N, Niparko JK. Complications of Temporal Bone. In: Flint PW, Haughey BH, Lund VJ, Niparko JK, Richardson MA, eds. *Cummings Otolaryngology: Head & Neck Surgery.* 5th ed. Philadelphia: Mosby Elsevier; 2010.

Send Orders of Reprints at reprints@benthamscience.net

# CHAPTER 4

## Hearing Loss

## Brian K. Reilly[1,*], Max Pusz[2] and Kenneth M. Grundfast[3]

[1]*George Washington University School of Medicine; Children's National Medical Center; Washington, D.C. USA;* [2]*Walter Reed National Military Medical Center Bethesda, Bethesda, Maryland and* [3]*Department of Otolaryngology-Head and Neck Surgery, Boston University School of Medicine, Boston, Massachusetts, USA*

**Abstract:** With the widespread utilization of universal newborn hearing screening during the past two decades, early detection of hearing impairment in children has improved markedly. This chapter provides an overview of early identification of childhood hearing impairment, methods used for early detection, common causes, and the various rehabilitative interventions both medical, surgical, and technological. A primary care physician who is knowledgeable about pediatric hearing impairment can play a key role in achieving the best possible outcome.

**Keywords:** Hearing loss, Hearing impairment, Universal Newborn Screening, Otitis media, Cochlear implant, BAHA, Otoacoustic emissions, ABR, Audiologic testing, Audiogram, Conductive, Sensorineural, Tympanometry, Hearing Aid, Deafness, Auditory Neuropathy, Ossicles, Connexin, Speech Therapy, Tympanostomy tube, Tympanoplasty.

## INTRODUCTION

Congenital hearing loss, which occurs in 2 to 4 per 1000 live births, is the most common birth disorder in newborns [1]. If an infant's hearing impairment is not detected early in life, then the affected child can encounter difficulty with acquiring speech and probably will experience problems with cognitive development and future academic performance. To avoid delays in detection of congenital hearing loss, universal newborn hearing screening has been implemented throughout the United States and in almost all developed countries.

*Address correspondence to Brian Reilly:** Children's National Medical Center, 111 Michigan Avenue, NW, Washington, D.C. 20010, USA; E-mail: breilly@cnmc.org

**Rahul K. Shah, Diego A. Preciado and George H. Zalzal (Eds)**

Normal hearing enables a child to acquire the "code of language" but, depending on the severity, hearing loss can impede and delay a child's ability to achieve important language milestones - from the baby's first few "coos" at age 6 months, to the infant's first words around 12 months, to the first sentences that occur by age 2, and to storytelling at age 4. The child who is delayed in developing speech is at risk for concomitant problems with communication and social behavior which can result in poor school performance and constrained social interactions. Research by the National Center for Hearing Assessment and Management (NCHAM) has shown that early detection and treatment for hearing loss for one child saves $400,000 in special education costs by the time that child graduates from high school [2].

The causes of childhood hearing loss are numerous and sometimes multifactorial. Congenital hearing impairment can be caused by intrauterine infection or a genetic mutation in the fetus. Hearing loss in early childhood can be caused by ear infections, viruses, ototoxic medications, cholesteatoma, or in rare instances, a neoplasm. Childhood hearing loss can be an isolated disorder or it can occur along with other abnormalities that are recognizable as a syndrome.

The prevalence of pediatric hearing loss increases to six per one thousand by the time a child is six years of age. This increase can be attributed to a combination of factors, including a delay in detection of a hearing loss that had been present at birth, genetic disorders that are characterized by onset of hearing loss beginning several years after birth, hearing impairment related to persistent middle ear effusion, and erosion of middle ear ossicles from cholesteatoma. Therefore, the parent and pediatrician should always watch for signs of hearing impairment and be ready to intervene with diagnostic testing if a child is delayed in developing speech or seems to have difficulty hearing.

A relevant guiding principle should be this: whenever a parent or caregiver voices the suspicion that a child is not hearing normally, that child should be considered to be hearing impaired until proven otherwise. If hearing loss is suspected, then that child should be evaluated by an audiologist who is accustomed to testing the hearing of children. The otolaryngologist (ENT doctor) works with the audiologists, speech therapists, and hearing aid dispensers to ensure that children reach their appropriate speech and linguistic potential and provides the critical link between pediatricians and families.

This chapter aims to provide pediatricians and family practitioners with information helpful for early detection and optimal management of hearing loss in young children.

## PATHOPHYSIOLOGY

Hearing loss is the most common congenital sensory impairment. Hearing thresholds assess the response of the listener to sound as it travels from the outer, to the middle and inner ear. Action potentials transmitted along the cochlear nerve from the inner ear to the auditory cortex provide for the brain's perception of sound. Any disruption along the auditory pathway can affect a child's ability to hear. Normal hearing in children is considered to be the ability to detect a sound at the level of 20 decibels or less. Hearing loss in the frequencies between 300 and 3000Hz, affect speech comprehension more than hearing loss at other frequencies.

## RISK FACTORS

It is estimated that there are 33 babies born every day with significant hearing loss, which is nearly 12,000 babies per year in the United States [3]. Risk factors for a child being born with an abnormal ability to hear include *in-utero* infections (*e.g.*, TORCH, as defined in Table **1**), post-natal infections associated with hearing loss, positive family history of permanent childhood sensorineural hearing loss, identification of a syndrome known to be associated with congenital or progressive hearing loss, severe hyperbilirubinemia requiring exchange transfusion, prematurity with birth weight less than 1800 grams, prolonged intubation, NICU admission, HIV+ status, and chronic or loud noise exposure (JCIH position statement 2000) [4].

**Table 1:** Perinatal Infections which Cause Hearing Loss

| T | Toxoplasmosis |
|---|---|
| O | Other Syphilis, HIV positive, Varicella-Zoster, Parvovirus B19 |
| R | Rubella |
| C | Cytomegalovirus |
| H | Herpes simplex Virus Type 2 |

## AUDIOLOGIC TESTING

Prompt audiologic testing is critical to making a diagnosis of childhood hearing loss as early as possible. Techniques used by audiologists to assess the hearing of young childen include: immittance testing, speech testing, behavioral observational audiometry, visual reinforcement audiometry, and play audiometry. An audiogram is obtained to determine the degree and/or severity of hearing loss as well as the frequency ranges most affected. Initial audiologic testing at birth involves otoacoustic emissions (OAEs) and/or auditory brainstem response (ABR) testing to assess hearing. Newborns with additional certain risk factors should always undergo screening ABR.

Older children with suspected hearing loss that have not undergone newborn hearing screening or have developed suspected hearing loss since their newborn hearing screen can undergo other forms of audiologic testing depending on age and cognitive development. Behavioral observational audiometry is used in very young children (less than 6 months) and is based on a child's reflexive response when a sound is presented, *i.e.*, startle or eye widening. Behavioral observational audiometry gives a gross estimate of hearing at best and should not be used to assume true hearing thresholds.

Generally, by the age of 6 months, children can be evaluated with visual reinforcement audiometry. Visual reinforcement audiometry uses "operant conditioning" in which the child is prompted or conditioned to turn his head in response to sound. The head turn is reinforced with an animated toy or other item of interest. Around the age of three years, conditioned play audiometry can be used to assess hearing. Play audiometry uses interactive games in which the child responds to sounds by performing a task such as stacking blocks. By 5 years of age, most children can participate in testing with standard audiometric techniques, similar to those used for an adult.

Speech testing enables an audiologist to determine an individual's speech awareness threshold or speech reception threshold, which is the softest sound level that elicits a response. Of note, speech testing can be incorporated into any of the above discussed behavioral assessment measures.

Immittance testing, or tympanometry, is used to assess eardrum mobility and provides information about the function of the middle ear. Immittance testing includes tympanometric findings, such as external auditory canal volume and acoustic reflex levels. It is helpful in detection of middle ear fluid as well as tympanic membrane perforations and retractions.

## Degree of Hearing Loss

Based on the results of the audiogram, a child's hearing loss is classified on two scales. First, the degree of hearing loss is diagnosed as mild, moderate, moderately-severe, severe, or profound.

The values that correspond to the degree of hearing loss are identified in Table **2**.

**Table 2:** Normal Hearing *versus* Degrees of Hearing Loss

| Normal Hearing | 0 to 20 dB HL |
| --- | --- |
| Mild Hearing Loss | 21 to 40 dB HL |
| Moderate Hearing Loss | 41 to 55 dB HL |
| Moderately Severe Loss | 56 to 70 dB HL |
| Severe Hearing Loss | 71 to 90 dB HL |
| Profound Hearing Loss | Greater than 90 dB HL |

## Hearing Loss Classifications

Hearing loss is classified as sensorineural, conductive, or mixed (a combination of sensorineural hearing loss and conductive hearing loss). Sensorineural hearing loss results when there has been damage to cochlear structures or the cochlear nerve. Conductive hearing loss occurs when there has been a loss of the mechanical transmission of sound along the pathway from the outer ear to the oval window. A blockage of sound anywhere from the ear canal, down the ossicular chain, to the cochlea causes conductive hearing loss.

There are several common causes of conductive hearing which include: 1) cerumen impaction 2) perforation of the tympanic membrane 3) middle ear fluid 4) fixation, erosion, or discontinuity of the ossicular chain from either a congenital abnormality or the sequela of significant ear infections. Even a mild to moderate conductive hearing loss may cause noticeable effect on speech and language development.

## INFANT AND CHILD SCREENING

Universal Newborn Hearing screening commenced in the 1990s and has facilitated the early detection of significant hearing loss in newborns, especially in children without risk factors. The goal of early screening is to identify hearing loss during the critical language acquisition window so that the child can be fitted with hearing aids or receive a cochlear implant as soon as the severity of a hearing impairment has been determined. In particular, the Joint Committee on Infant Hearing recommends screening for hearing loss by 1 month, audiologic diagnosis by 3 months, and enrollment in early intervention services by six months.

Otoacoustic emissions (OAEs) are used in the newborn hearing screening test and identify a hearing threshold of at least 30 dB HL. Either DPOAEs (distortion product otoacoustic emissions) or TEOAEs (transient evoked otoacoustic emissions) are used, as protocols vary depending on the audiology site/testing center. The outer hair cells of the cochlea emit OAEs, which are then detected and measured *via* sensitive microphones within the device. Newborn nurseries, which perform testing for otoacoustic emissions, demonstrate high sensitivity but low specificity. OAEs have a reported sensitivity of 90-100% and a specificity range of 82-84% [5-7].

The OAE screening test is valuable because it is simple, inexpensive, non-invasive and objective (does not require any input from the patient). This test has some limitations as it is unable to detect retrocochlear lesions or auditory neuropathies. However, OAEs alone do not lead to a specific diagnosis. For every 1,000 babies that are screened there is a 1.2 percent referral rate for further testing. Of those 12 infants who are further tested, 3 will have a sensorineural hearing loss, 1 to 2 per 1000 will have transient conductive hearing loss, and 7 to 8 will have normal hearing.

Recently, Automated Auditory Brainstem Response (AABR) testing has become available as an addition to Universal Newborn Hearing Screening protocols. Similar to OAE testing, AABR uses clicks and evaluates the electrical response of the peripheral and central auditory system up to the level of the brainstem. Usually only those patients with certain risk factors (NICU stay greater than 5 days, hyperbilirubinemia, low birth weight, extreme prematurity (<28 weeks), hypoxia, anoxia, prolonged assisted ventilation), congenital brain anomalies, certain demyelenating syndromes, *etc.*) will undergo AABR screening as well as OAE screening. The purpose of the AABR is to rule out auditory neuropathy

(AN), as an infant with a devastating hearing loss *via* AN will likely pass a simple OAE screening.

If the OAE or AABR screening tests are abnormal, further evaluation with a diagnostic conventional auditory brainstem response (ABR), also known as brainstem auditory evoked response testing (BAER) should be performed. Diagnostic ABR enables the audiologist to identify the specific degree and frequency range of an existing hearing loss. ABR assesses the hearing pathway from the cochlea to the auditory brainstem. ABR test essentially measures neuroelectric potentials from the auditory nerve to the brainstem, similar to how an EKG measures the electric potentials of the heart. ABR is particularly helpful in numerous infants and children who are unable to participate in behavioral audiometry.

Infants with newborn screening exams that are within normal limits, but who have other risk factors associated with delayed onset hearing loss should undergo hearing evaluation every six months for the first three years of life. As children become school age, most will undergo regular hearing screenings during grade school.

## CAUSES OF HEARING LOSS

### Hereditary Hearing Loss

Hereditary hearing loss can be separated into disorders caused by autosomal recessive and autosomal dominant patterns of inheritance. The majority of genetic hearing loss is autosomal recessive (up to 80%); the remainder is autosomal dominant (around 15%) or sex-linked and mitochondrial inheritance (around 5%).

Childhood hearing loss can also be separated into non-syndromic hearing loss, in which hearing loss is the only abnormality, and syndromic hearing loss, in which hearing loss is associated with other genetic abnormalities. Between 10-20% of congenital hearing loss is syndromic.

### Genetic Testing

There are over 40 different genes that have been found to cause autosomal recessive hearing loss. The most common genetic etiology of hearing loss is the autosomal recessive GJB2 gene, which produces the protein connexin 26. Connexin 26 is a gap junction protein which is involved in transport in potassium in the stria vascularis of the cochlea. Connexin mutation is the most often cause of non-syndromic, genetic hearing loss. GJB2 hearing loss is attributed to 20% of all genetic hearing loss. The hearing loss is present either at birth or early during infancy. Connexin testing is helpful because the hearing loss associated with it does not usually worsen with time. Additional gap junction proteins such as connexin 30 may also contribute to the hearing loss.

## Syndromic Hearing Loss

Syndromic hearing loss occurs when hearing loss is associated with at least one other detectable congenital abnormality. The hearing loss can be sensorineural, conductive or mixed. Children that have hearing loss should be closely evaluated for any other genetic abnormalities because hearing loss is generally the first and most apparent finding of the syndrome.

### Autosomal Recessive Syndromes

*Jervell Lange-Neilson syndrome* is a rare syndrome that affects potassium channels causing sensorineural hearing loss associated with a cardiac conduction defect. The electrocardiogram (EKG) shows a prolonged QT interval. It can present with syncope. The degree of hearing loss can vary, but is usually severe to profound. A simple screening EKG should be performed in patients with congenital severe to profound hearing loss so as to detect this condition and prevent an arrhythmia which can lead to sudden death.

*Pendred syndrome (PS)* includes sensorineural hearing loss and abnormal iodine metabolism. Children with PS can develop goiter in early adolescence. The SLC26A4 gene produces the protein pendrin that is responsible for the transport of iodine and chloride. The hearing loss can be profound at birth or progressive. The syndrome commonly includes an enlarged vestibular aqueduct and cochlear dysplasia. Previously an abnormal perchlorate test was used to detect thyroid dysfunction. Currently, genetic testing can detect the SLC26A4 gene and lead to diagnosis.

Children with PS may also have an enlarged vestibular aqueduct (EVA) independent of Pendred syndrome (Fig. **1**). Hearing loss associated with an EVA is usually sensorineural, but can be conductive or mixed. Patients with an EVA are at risk for sudden hearing loss after trauma, possibly due to bleeding into the endolymphatic sac. Therefore, it is recommended that patients with EVA refrain from activities such as contact sports in which the likelihood of head trauma is increased. The cause of the conductive component of the hearing loss is due to the third window effect whereby the abnormal communication between the dilated endolymphatic sac and enlarged endolymphatic duct acts as the 'third window' for sound conductance.

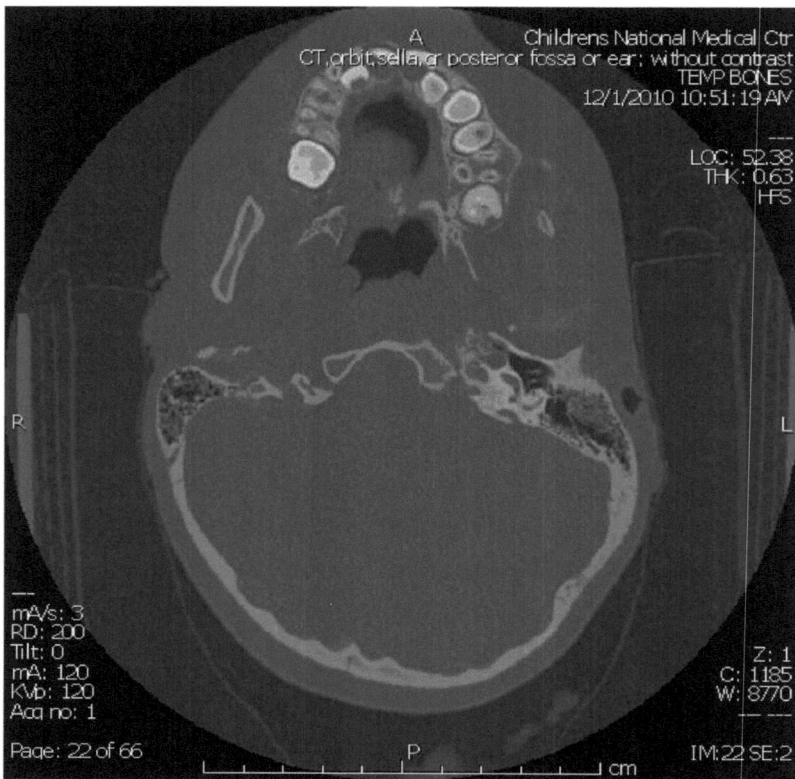

**Figure 1:** Left Enlarged vestibular aqueduct.

*Alport syndrome* is a progressive multi-system condition that includes chronic glomerulonephritis, leading to end-stage kidney disease, and hearing loss as a co-morbidity. The hearing loss does not occur until late childhood or early adult life. A hearing loss always accompanies renal involvement and routine urinalysis will detect abnormal levels of proteinuria.

*Usher syndrome* is the leading causes of deaf blindness in the United States of America. Children with significant hearing loss should undergo ophthamologic evaluation. The syndrome consists of retinitis pigmentosa and sensorineural hearing loss. There are three main types of Usher syndrome: Usher type I consists of bilateral profound hearing loss and absent vestibular function, Usher type II consists of moderate hearing loss and normal vestibular function, Usher type III consists of progressive hearing loss and variable vestibular function.

## Autosomal Dominant Syndromes

*Branchio-oto-renal syndrome* consists of conductive, sensorineural or mixed hearing loss, and branchial derived abnormalities such as ear pits and renal abnormalities from minor dysplasia to renal agenesis. Cochlear abnormalities are also commonly seen.

*Treacher-Collins syndrome* is also known as mandibulo-facial-dysostosis and includes craniofacial abnormalities combined with microtia and ossicular chain malformations that are associated with conductive hearing loss. In small numbers of patients, both sensorineural hearing loss and vestibular dysfunction can be seen.

*Waardenburg syndrome* results in unilateral or bilateral sensorineural hearing loss with pigment abnormalities such as a white forelock, craniofacial abnormalities including dystopia canthorum, and commonly an enlarged vestibular aqueduct.

## Conductive Hearing Loss

The causes of conductive hearing loss can range from the simple cerumen impaction to complete occlusion of the ear canal from aural atresia, with absent external auditory canal. However, the most common cause of conductive hearing loss in children is from middle ear effusion, typically caused by otitis media. The hearing loss is expected to have a complete resolution after the effusion (fluid) resolves. In 90% of children the effusion will resolve after 3 months. Otitis media with effusion (OME) that persists longer than this and results in speech delay may require tympanostomy tubes.

Another cause of conductive hearing loss in children is cholesteatoma. Cholesteatoma can occur from an embryologic rest of squamous cells that become implanted in the middle ear during gestation, or from severe eustachian tube dysfunction causing a retraction of the tympanic membrane. A cholesteatoma is a collection of bone destroying squamous cells that have been trapped in the middle ear. The squamous cells produce destructive enzymes and biofilms, which untreated can lead to local destruction of middle ear structures, particularly the incudostapedial joint connection.

## ADDITIONAL EVALUATIONS AND WORK-UP

There are important medical reasons to identify hearing loss and determine the prognosis for further hearing deterioration in every child with impairment. Comprehensive evaluations enable the development of a proper management plan for the child aimed at helping the child to reach his or her maximal potential for education and life achievement while, at the same time, assisting the family in coping with the difficulties encountered in raising a hearing impaired child. After all, families of a hearing impaired child often need counseling to find the most appropriate setting for their child's pre-school and primary school education. Therefore, early and comprehensive screening tests are of immense value.

### Congenital Hearing Loss

A history of prematurity is also an important part of the perinatal history. Significant bilateral hearing loss is ten times more prevalent in infants that have been in the Neonatal Intensive Care Unit for more than 3 days [8]. Accordingly, the Joint Committee on Infant Hearing recommended, in their 2007 position statement, that all neonates that are in the intensive care unit for more than 5 days undergo hearing screening with auditory brainstem response (ABR) testing.

All infants who have failed their hearing screening test and have undergone formal audiologic testing that has proven hearing loss should undergo a more extensive workup to identify the causes of the hearing loss. The commonly recommended workup includes: GJB2 genetic testing, CT scan of the temporal bones, thyroid studies, electrocardiogram, an ophthalmologic evaluation, and a urinalysis and possible renal ultrasound. MRI scans are increasingly valued and confirm hypoplasia or aplasia of the VIII cochlear nerve divisions.

After a child has been found to have congenital hearing loss, the "on-going" evaluation entails a thorough review of the medical findings, physical exam findings, and radiographic findings. Physical exam findings in particular can lead to identification of syndromic causes of hearing loss. Consultations are often made for the patient to see a geneticist, ophthalmologist, and otolaryngologist.

## Imaging

### *Computed Tomography*

Children identified with hearing loss on a screening examination that has been confirmed with ABR most often will have radiological imaging of the temporal bone and adjacent brainstem using a non-contrast computed tomography (CT) scan of the temporal bones. The CT scan can provide excellent images showing the structural integrity of the auditory system within the temporal bones at the base of the skull. The radiologist examines the internal auditory canal, vestibular aqueduct, the cochlea, the vestibule and semicircular canals, the ossicular chain, oval and round windows, as well as the tympanic membrane and external auditory canal.

### *Mangetic Resonance Imanging*

Magnetic resonance imaging (MRI) of the temporal bone and internal auditory canal is particularly useful for evaluating possible cholesteatoma, cholesterol granuloma, and cochlear fibrosis and ossification. Absent cochlear nerves (agenesis or hypogenesis) are able to be detected. These findings are critical and must be determined before suggesting any surgical intervention, such as cochlear implantation.

## TREATMENT

## Conductive Hearing Loss

The great majority of causes of conductive hearing loss can be treated surgically with an improvement in hearing. For example, conductive hearing loss caused by middle ear effusion (OME) is usually self-limited, but if prolonged can be easily alleviated with myringotomy and tympanostomy tube placement. Perforations of the tympanic membrane can be caused from infection, trauma or as a complication of surgery such as ear tubes. The perforation leads to a conductive hearing loss due to two mechanisms, loss of amplification of the tympanic membrane and sound arriving at the oval and round windows simultaneously.

Closure of the perforation *via* tympanoplasty repair will often return the hearing to near pre-perforation levels.

Congenital ossicular fixation, which most commonly involves the malleus, results in conductive hearing loss due to loss of normal sound transmission through the middle ear ossicles. Treatment requires middle ear exploration with ossiculoplasty or amplification with hearing aids.

Cholesteatomas can disrupt the ossicular chain and reduce transmission of sound to the middle ear causing conductive hearing loss. Once the presence of cholesteatoma has been identified clinically, a CT scan must be performed to determine the extent of disease in the middle ear and possible spread into the mastoid. A tympanomastoidectomy depending on the extent of disease is usually necessary to remove all of the squamous cell debris from the middle ear and mastoid. If left untreated, the cholesteatoma will continue to grow and erode critical middle ear structures such as the ossicles, cochlea, and mastoid bone.

Cholesteatoma and chronic suppurative otitis media, which are more rare in the antibiotic era can also be treated by performing a mastoidectomy alone as an isolated single procedure. A surgical mastoidectomy is a procedure in which the surgeon drills the mastoid bone into the middle ear space to eliminate the middle ear and mastoid disease. In some situations a "second look" procedure is recommended to confirm that all of the cholesteatoma has been completely removed from the middle ear and mastoid. When the cholesteatoma has caused damage to or destruction of the middle ear bones (middle ear ossicles) resulting in a conductive hearing loss, then a procedure to reconstruct the bones known as an ossiculoplasty can be performed to restore the child's hearing.

## Sensorineural Hearing Loss

Any child that has been found to have sensorineural hearing loss must undergo a workup such as the evaluation listed above. In addition, there are some young children and adolescents who may develop an autoimmune sensorineural hearing loss (AISHL). AISHL sometimes respond to oral steroids, such as prednisolone, or transtympanic injections of prednisone. A serologic work-up can include ESR, CRP, CBC, Rheumatoid Factors, and anti-neutrophil antibodies (ANA) levels. When there are no medical contra-indications, the child can undergo a hearing aid trial.

## HEARING AIDS

Children with mild to moderate/moderate to severe hearing loss should be fitted with hearing aids as early as possible. Hearing aids can provide improvement up to a level of 60dB. When levels exceed 60dB, hearing aids can actually become uncomfortable due to the pressure against the tympanic membrane. There are multiple different styles of hearing aids available but the best type of hearing aid for young children is a hearing aid that sits behind the ear (a.k.a. behind-the-ear hearing aid). In school age children with mild hearing loss, an FM transmitter unit may be used. This FM unit consists of a microphone worn by the teacher and a receiver and amplifier worn by the student. Preferential seating in the front of the classroom can also be beneficial.

The hearing aids should be fitted bilaterally if the hearing loss is bilateral because it has been shown that children fitted with monaural hearing aids, as compared to children with binaural hearing aids, have significantly worse speech recognition scores [9]. After hearing aids have been fitted, speech therapy is recommended because children develop speech by mimicking sounds they hear.

There have been major advances in hearing aids. They now connect to FM systems and MP3 players. Hearing aids can be digitally programmed, configured to an individual's specific hearing loss, and adjusted to filter out background noise. Current models have become small in size making them able to fit comfortably behind the ear or in the ear canal (Fig. **2**). All patients should get medical clearance for hearing aids to rule out possible surgical or medical pathology.

## RECENT ADVANCEMENTS

### Cochlear Implantation

For those children who have bilateral severe-to-profound sensorineural hearing loss and therefore, do not benefit from hearing aids, cochlear implantation may be a viable treatment option. Young children (12 to 24 months) are candidates for a cochlear implant if they have profound hearing loss (>90dB), lack of speech development and no benefit with the use of hearing aids. Children older than 24 months are candidates if they have a hearing loss greater than 70dB, with speech discrimination score less than 20%, and a hearing in noise (HINT) scores of less than 50%. The children should also have no medical contraindications to implantation. Post-meningitic onset of hearing loss may lead to deafness and requires urgent evaluation and treatment and is an indication for early cochlear implantation. There is a current trend toward implantation as early as 6 months at certain centers.

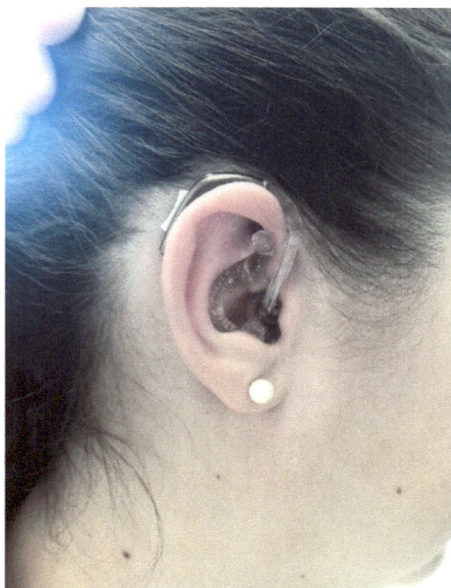

**Figure 2:** Behind the Ear Hearing Aid.

A specially trained committee of audiologists, speech therapists, and otolaryngologists meets regularly to discuss candidacy for cochlear implantation in those infants who meet the criterion. A cochlear implant evaluation entails precise audiologic assessment, radiologic examination of the cochlea and Cranial Nerve VIII by MRI and CT scan, with surgical evaluation by an otolaryngologist, and speech therapy assessment. The evaluation should also include an analysis of the social and family structure.

To start, candidates are recommended to undergo a hearing aid trial to test whether hearing aids are sufficient or whether an implant may be more beneficial. A hearing aid trial is the standard of care before cochlear implantation unless there is evidence of progressive ossification of the cochlea from meningitis, which can make cochlear implantation difficult or even impossible. Although, it is recommended that children undergo implantation at age >12 months, post-meningitic patients with profound hearing loss may be implanted prior to 12 months of age due the risk of ossification of the cochlea.

Surgical candidacy is then determined by confirming that the anatomy is favorable to implantation. MRI and/or CT scanning are needed to assess anatomy and to evaluate for cochlear, vestibular, and facial nerve locations, as well as to confirm the presence of the auditory nerve (CN VIII).

Cochlear implants are implanted into the scala tympani of the cochlea and stimulate the spiral ganglion neurons. The units are implanted beneath the scalp, the receiver is held in place on the outside of the skin by a magnet, and the processor is behind the ear (Fig. **3**). After patients have undergone cochlear implantation, they need close follow up with an audiologist specially trained in cochlear implantation for activation and programming as well as speech therapy.

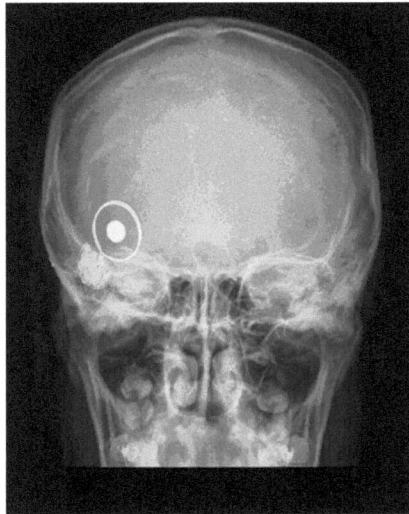

**Figure 3:** Cochlear Implant in Position.

Cochlear implantation can be performed as young as 6 months of age. Implants are FDA approved for children aged 12 months or older with profound bilateral hearing loss (Fig. **4**) and for adults with similar hearing loss who demonstrate limited benefit from hearing aid use as demonstrated by speech perception test scores.

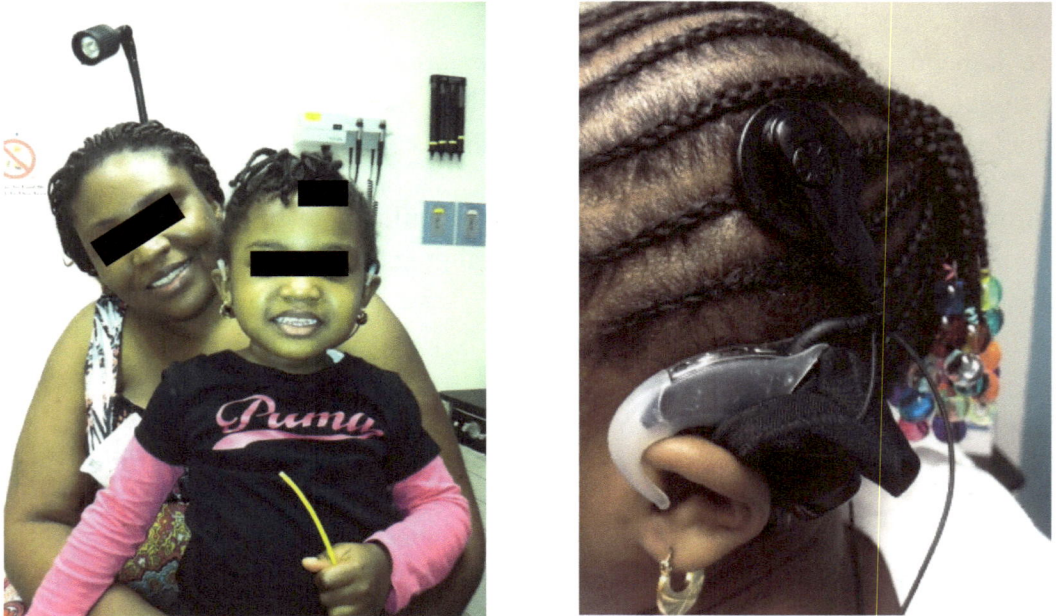

**Figure 4:** Bilateral Cochlear Implant Recipient.

Cochlear implants were FDA approved in 1984 for adults and 1990 for children. Unlike a hearing aid that only amplifies sound, a cochlear implant functions like the actual human cochlea and transduces mechanical sound energy into an electric impulse. It has been shown that children with cochlear implants have nearly the same language development as children with normal hearing [10]. Generally, the younger a child is implanted the better the speech and language outcome.

More recently there has been an increasing trend towards bilateral cochlear implantation in children. It has been shown that children with bilateral implantation have better speech recognition in noise as well as better sound localization [11]. Bilateral recipients also show an advantage regarding speech intelligibility [12]. The William House Cochlear Implant Society has issued a formal position statement in support of bilateral implantation [13]. The current trend is to implant an infant as young as possible to provide maximal benefit.

**Bone-Anchored Hearing Implant System (BAHA)**

In pediatric patients with conductive hearing loss, who have mixed hearing loss or single sided deafness (unilateral profound sensorineural hearing loss), a bone-anchored hearing system may be used instead of other hearing aids. The indications for patients with conductive hearing loss are a near maximal conductive hearing loss of >45dB with less than a 35dB sensorineural component of hearing loss.

The BAHA implant consists of a two-stage procedure in children. The first stage is the implantation of the titanium fixture in the temporal bone. The second stage of the procedure occurs after a three-month period, which allows time for the osseointegration of the implant to occur. The second stage involves thinning the subcutaneous tissue around the fixture, placing a skin graft, and attaching the abutment. Once the graft has healed after 3-6 months, the transducer (vibrating hearing bone ossicilator) is attached to the abutment and transmits sound to the functioning cochlea.

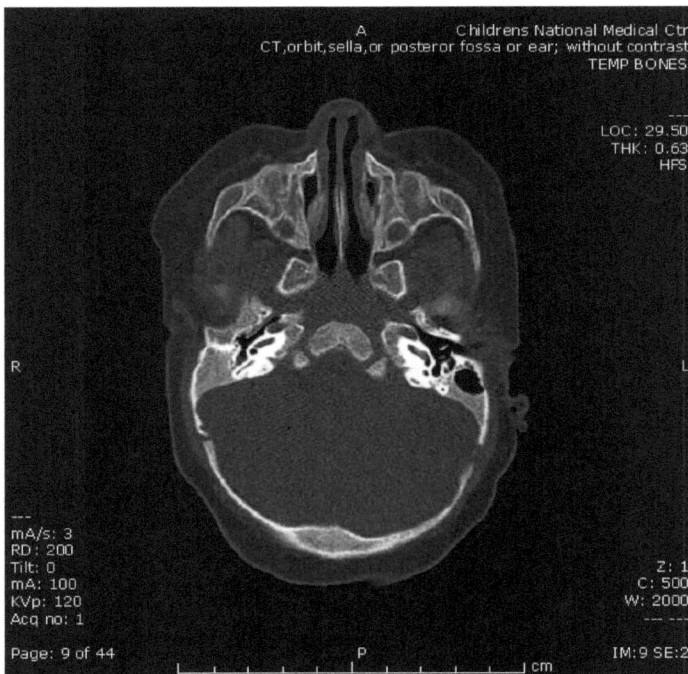

**Figure 5:** Right Sided Congenital Atresia.

BAHAs are currently FDA approved for children older than 5 years of age. Children younger than 5 years of age can use the BAHA soft band, which is a non-implanted BAHA device worn on the head with an elastic headband. This can be particularly useful in children with unilateral or bilateral aural atresia or those with Treacher Collins (Fig. **5**). Patients treated with the BAHA soft band with bilateral aural atresia have improved speech and language outcomes [14].

## CONCLUSION

With the widespread utilization of universal newborn hearing screening during the past two decade, early detection of hearing impairment in children has improved markedly. Therefore, it is increasingly important for primary care physicians to be familiar with the expectations for early identification of childhood hearing impairment, methods used for early detection, common causes and the array of rehabilitative interventions that can be offered to assist the hearing impaired child.

A primary care physician who is knowledgeable about early child hearing impairment can play a key role in achieving for the child and the family best possible outcome even in the cases of severe hearing impairment or deafness.

## ACKNOWLEDGEMENT

Declared none.

## CONFLICT OF INTEREST

The author(s) confirm that this chapter content has no conflict of interest.

## REFERENCES

[1]　Boyle CA, Decoufle P, Yeargin-Allsopp M. Prevalence and health impact of developmental disabilities in US children. Pediatrics 1994;93:399-403.
[2]　National Center for Hearing Assessment and Management. http://www.infanthearing.org/
[3]　Centers for Disease Control and Prevention. National Center for Birth Defects and Developmental Disabilities, Early Hearing Detection and Intervention Program. http://www.cdc.gov/ncbddd/ehdi/default.htm.
[4]　Committee on Infant Hearing.Joint Committee on Infant Hearing 2000 position statement. Pediatrics 2000;106:4:798-817.
[5]　Maxon AB, White KR, Behrens TR, *et al.* Referral rates and cost efficiency in a universal newborn hearing screening program using transient evoked otoacoustic emissions. J Am AcadAudiol 1995;6:271-7.
[6]　Kennedy CR, Kimm L, Dees DC, *et al.* Otoacoustic emissions and auditory brainstem responses in the newborn. Arch Dis Child 1991;66:1124-9.
[7]　Salata JA, Jacobson JT, Strasnick B. Distortion-product otoacoustic emissions hearing screening in high-risk newborns. Otolaryngol Head Neck Surg 1998;118:37-43.

[8]    Task Force on Newborn and Infant Hearing. Newborn and Infant Hearing Loss: Detection and Intervention. Pediatrics 1999;103:2:527-530.

[9]    Gelfand SA, Silman S. Apparent auditory deprivation in children: implications of monaural *versus* binaural amplification. J Am AcadAudiol 1993;4:313-8.

[10]   Svirsky MA, Robbins AM, Kirk KI, *et al.* Language development in profoundly deaf children with cochlear implants. PsycholSci 2000;11:153-8.

[11]   Lovett RE, Kitterick PT, Hewitt CE, *et al.* Bilateral or unilateral cochlear implantation for deaf children: an observational study. Arch Dis Child 2010;95:107-12.

[12]   Litovsky RY, Johnstone PM, Godar SP. Benefits of bilateral cochlear implants and/or hearing aids in children. Int J Audiol 2006;45Suppl 1:S78-91.

[13]   Balkany T, Hodges A, Telischi F, *et al.* William House Cochlear Implant Study Group: position statement on bilateral cochlear implantation. Otol Neurotol 2008; 107-8.

[14]   Verhagen CV, Hol MK, Coppens-Schellekens W, *et al.* The BahaSoftband. A new treatment for young children with bilateral congenital aural atresia.Int J PediatrOtorhinolaryngol 2008;72:1455-9.

*Send Orders of Reprints at reprints@benthamscience.net*

# CHAPTER 5

## Adenoiditis/Sinusitis

### Charles A. Elmaraghy[*]

*Department of Otolaryngology, Nationwide Children's Hospital, The Ohio State University College of Medicine, OH, USA*

**Abstract:** Pediatric sinusitis and adenoiditis are common conditions that are difficult to distinguish. Disruption of normal sinus physiology can lead to sinusitis and conditions such as asthma, GERD, cystic fibrosis, and ciliary dysmotility may contribute to the condition of chronic sinusitis. Diagnosis of adenoiditis and sinusitis may be difficult and necessitate more work-up than physical exam. The firstline treatment of both conditions requires antibiotics but may require adjuvant treatment such as nasal steroids nasal saline and targeted therapy towards any contributing conditions such as allergies or GERD. Evaluation involves physical exam, nasal endoscopy, and in patients recalcitrant to treatment, CT scans. Failure of medical therapy may necessitate surgical intervention.

**Keywords:** Sinusitis, adenoiditis, sinus surgery, adenoidectomy, cystic fibrosis, mucociliary, adenoidectomy, nasal polyp, otolaryngology, otolaryngologist, pediatric sinusitis, nasal discharge, GERD, sinus, ethmoid sinus, maxillary sinus, endscopic, rhinorrhea, nasal congestion, URI.

## INTRODUCTION

Pediatric sinusitis and adenoiditis are common entities encountered by pediatricians and family practitioners. Sinusitis is the 5th most common reason for pediatric patients to visit their practitioner and obtain an antibiotic. Upper respiratory infections are largely viral, however, 5-13% of viral URIs are complicated by bacterial sinusitis of which 5-10% do not respond to initial treatment [1]. Although these are common entities, the diagnosis may be subtle and it may be difficult to know when to refer to a specialist for management. The goal of this chapter is to review the basics of these disease processes and the current management.

## ANATOMY

The nasal cavity and sinuses develop throughout childhood. The sinuses are areas

*Address correspondence to Charles A. Elmaraghy:** Interim Chief, Assistant Professor, Department of Otolaryngology, Nationwide Children's Hospital, The Ohio State University College of Medicine, OH. USA; Tel: 614-722-6804; Fax: 614-722-6609; E-mail: charles.elmaraghy@osumc.edu

of pneumatization in the skull. At birth, the maxillary and ethmoid sinuses are present but not fully developed. The frontal and sphenoid sinuses develop later with the frontal sinus developing last with changes occurring until around age 20 years (Fig. **1**).

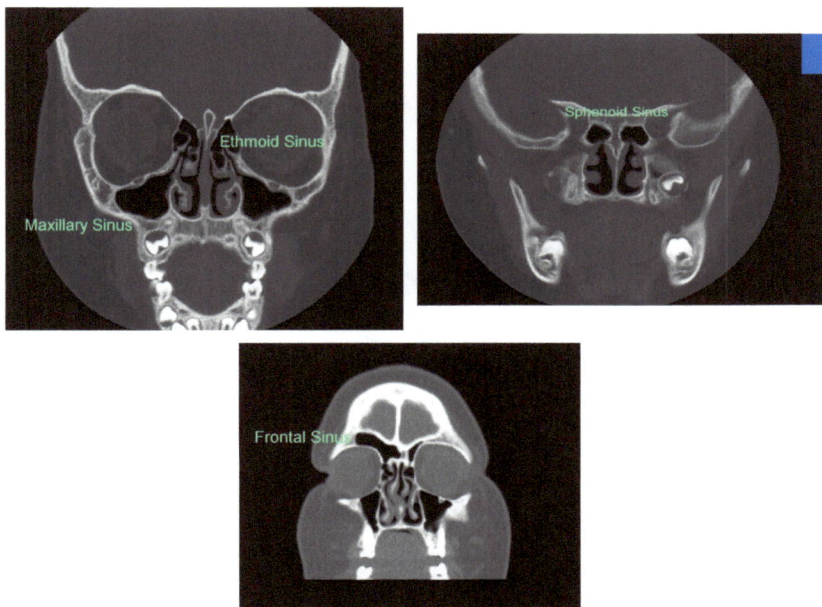

**Figure 1:** Normal Coronal CT Scans of the Sinuses.

## PHYSIOLOGY

The purposes of the sinuses are to humidify air circulating through the nasal cavity. The sinuses also produce mucous, which has important antibacterial properties and essentially acts as a physiologic filtration system for pathogens and other environmental agents. Normal mucous is dependent on mucociliary flow throughout the nasal cavity. Mucociliary flow refers to the constant circulation of mucous through the sinus cavities and nasal cavity. The nasal cavity and sinus cavities are lined by pseudostratified columnar respiratory epithelium. The significance of this is the ciliated nature of these cells. These cells are responsible for the movement of mucous. Mucous does not drain in a gravity dependent fashion in the sinuses. Each sinus has a specific ostium, or opening, through which mucous drains. The ciliated cells circulate mucous in a very organized fashion towards the ostium of the sinus cavity where it drains. To have healthy sinuses, mucociliary flow through non-obstructed sinuses is the defining principle (Fig. **2**).

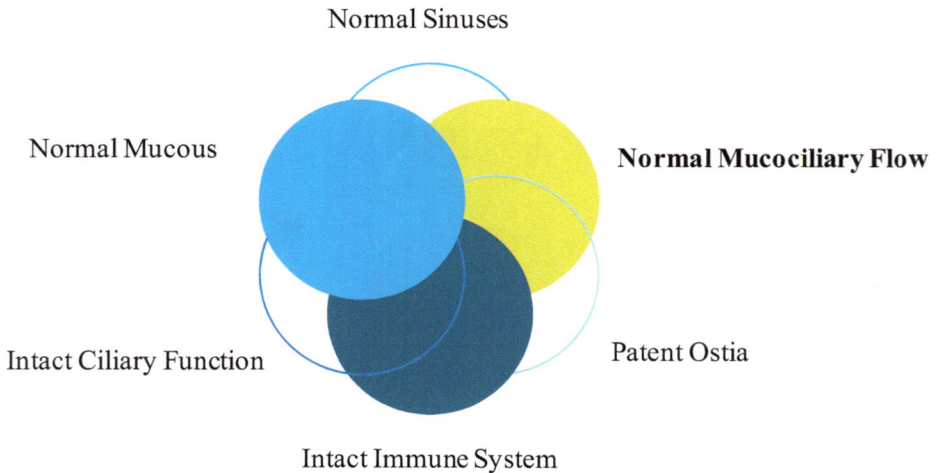

Normal Sinuses

Normal Mucous                                    **Normal Mucociliary Flow**

Intact Ciliary Function                                    Patent Ostia

Intact Immune System

**Figure 2:** Summary of Components of Normal Sinus Function.

The adenoid is a patch of tissue located in the naso-pharynx. It is a part of an aggregated of lymphoid tissue in the head and neck known as Waldeyer's ring. Lingual and palatine tonsils, posterior pharyngeal lymphoid tissues and the adenoid comprise the ring. The lymphoid tissue functions in as part of mucosal immunity and produce Immunoglobin G and A. The adenoid's location in the nasopharynx makes it a difficult structure to visualize as it can not be viewed directly. The adenoid is located in close proximity to the Eustachian tube orifice. The adenoid typically peaks in size from ages 2 to 4 years and typically regresses in size throughout adolescence.

## SYMPTOMATOLOGY

Symptoms of adenoiditis and sinusitis are virtually indistinguishable. Both share commons symptoms of nasal congestion, purulent, rhinorrhea, halitosis, nasal obstruction and longer duration of symptoms than the average URI. Upper respiratory viral infections and allergy symptoms can mimic sinusitis and adenoiditis, however, there are some distinguishing characteristics. Viral URIs may have fever associated with it but rarely last longer than 10 days, typically do not have halitosis associated with it, and not associated with dental pain. Allergy symptoms typically are clear rhinorrhea, never associated with fever, and do not have concomitant halitosis or dental pain. Distinguishing adenoiditis from sinusitis is not easily done on clinical grounds alone. Adenoid issues may be manifested more with nasal obstruction and snoring, although this is not always the case. The adenoid tissue may be chronically infected without severe hypertrophy. Severe adenoid hypertrophy will present with nasal obstruction and snoring is a common symptom. Chronic mouth breathing is also a known symptom of adenoid hypertrophy.

## PREDISPOSING FACTORS

Predisposing factors for inflammatory/infectious nasal and sinus issues are numerous. One of the more common predisposing factors is frequent viral upper respiratory tract infections. Children typically contract 6-10 viral URIs per year and this number can be much higher if the child attends daycare. Currently 30% of children in the United States attend daycare and this triples the odds of physician diagnosed sinusitis and problematic nasal drainage [1] Viruses can decrease mucociliary flow, increase edema of the sinus ostia, cause adenoid hypertrophy, and at the molecular level, increase expression of receptors that cause bacterial adherence.

An important predisposing factor for sinusitis and nasal problems in pediatric patients is the exposure to second-hand cigarette smoke. Tobacco smoke exposure promotes mucous stasis in the nasal cavity by impairing ciliary movement.

Asthma and allergies also are predisposing co-morbid conditions for sinusitis and nasal problems in pediatrics. Asthma is the most common co-morbidity in patients admitted to the hospital with a diagnosis of sinusitis [2]. The mechanism of naso-pulmonary interaction include aspiration of infected sinus secretions, vagal stimulation from constant nasal irritation resulting in bronchospasm, nasal obstruction leading to drying of distal airways, and circulating inflammatory mediatiors from bacterial toxins and nasal stimulation causing lower pulmonary symptoms. The airway from the nasal passages to the distal alveoli are related and co-dependent. This interaction has been termed the "unified airway". Allergies also potentiate nasal and sinus problems. This is typically an Ig E mediated process that increases tissue edema and mucous production. The result of this is to impair mucociliary function.

Gastro-esophageal reflux disease is another co-morbidity that has been implicated in the pathogenesis of pediatric nasal and sinus problems. Reflux can reach the level of the nasopharynx and the mucosal irritation and edema. Clinical improvement has been achieved in some recalcitrant chronic sinusitis patients with aggressive reflux treatment [3].

Patients with cystic fibrosis have a very high incidence of abnormal sinus CT scans (Fig. **3**). Nasal polyp disease in a child raises suspicion for cystic fibrosis and should be thoroughly worked up. The thick, tenacious, inspissated secretions common to cystic fibrosis lead to nasal and sinus disease. The microbiology of cystic fibrosis sinusitis is typically *Pseudomonas* or *Staphlococcus.* Surgical treatment of cystic fibrosis nasal and sinus disease is indicated with nasal obstruction secondary to polyps and bone erosion from sinus disease. There is some controversy as to the effect of sinus surgery on pulmonary function tests in CF patients. Retrospective literature have shown modest effects on PFT's [4].

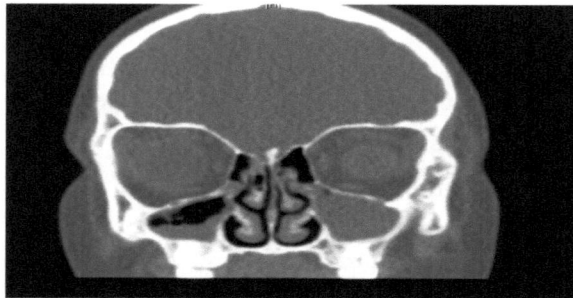

**Figure 3:** Abnormal CT Scan Revealing Opacification of Sinuses.

Ciliary motility issues can manifest with nasal and sinus problems. This can occur as a primary anomaly or secondary to infectious or environmental insult. The suprastructure of the cilia can be missing a critical component and the most common is absence of the dynein side arm. This results in a non-functional cilia. Infections and cigarette smoke can cause a secondary impairment of the cilia. The net result is stagnant mucous which can serve as an environment for pathogenic bacteria. Other issues with primary ciliary dyskinesia can be dextrocardia, male infertility, recurrent upper and lower respiratory tract infections.

In general, sinusitis and adenoiditis are easily treatable conditions that respond to conventional treatment as outlined below. However, chronic nasal problems may occur, and specifically with sinusitis, may be recalcitrant to treatment. The chronic nature of sinusitis in pediatric patients has been theorized to be due to an osteomyelitis model of pathology and/or biofilms.

In the osteomyelitis model, Kennedy *et al.* found evidence at the microscopic level of inflammation within the bone in specimens taken from the ethmoid bone during sinus surgery [5]. In addition, evidence of bone remodeling with increased fibrosis was noted in the specimens. This supports the observation of sinusitis requiring longer treatment courses with antibiotics due to poor penetration within the bone.

Biofilms are a topic of interest with regards to bacteriology and treatment of infections. Biofilms are colonies of bacteria surviving within a polysaccharide matrix. Their role in sinusitis is currently unknown, however, the resilience of biofilms to antibiotics may account for the chronic nature of some sinus infections. In addition, the electron microscopy of adenoid tissue has shown presence of bacteria existing in biofilms [6].

## DIAGNOSIS AND TREATMENT

Diagnosis of pediatric sinusitis and adenoiditis may be difficult as these structures are not directly visualized. On physical exam, thick, purulent rhinorrhea may be noted. The inferior turbinates may be hypertrophic and evidence of a post-nasal drip can sometimes be seen. It should be noted whether the child is able to breathe comfortably through the nares or if nasal obstruction is present. The widened midface and mouth breathing seen with adenoid hypertrophy is often referred to as "adenoid facies". Often, middle ear effusions can be seen with an enlarged adenoid.

A more extensive workup of sinusitis and adenoiditis should proceed after reasonable treatment has been achieved. Maximal medical therapy is often referred to, however, it is not defined. The American Academy of Pediatrics guidelines from 2001 recommend treatment of sinusitis to extend 7 days following the resolution of symptoms. The pencillins and cephalosporins are thought to be first-line antibiotic treatment with macrolides used for penicillin allergy. Fluoroquinolones are not thought to be first line for pediatric nasal infections. The duration of antibiotic treatment for sinusitis/adenoiditis may need to be 14-21 days for complete resolution of symptoms.

Adjunct medications in the treatment of sinusitis and adenoiditis may be helpful. Nasal saline is an often overlooked treatment in pediatrics. Nasal saline promotes normal mucocililary function and can often give symptomatic relief from troublesome rhinorrrhea. Compliance may be an issue in pediatric patients. The role of topical and systemic steroids in acute sinusitis is likely limited in the pediatric population. In pediatric patients without nasal polyp disease, there is likely no significant benefit in use of topical or systemic steroids in acute illness. Antihistamines and allergy medication in the absence of known allergy disease also have limited role. Currently, topical antibiotics have gained some popularity despite evidence suggesting poor penetration into the sinuses. Topical antibiotic rinses in the without prior sinus surgery do not have a role in the treatment of acute sinusitis and adenoiditis.

In patients that are unresponsive to treatment or have frequent episodes of sinusitis and adenoiditis, imaging is necessary. In younger patients or in patients with suspected adenoiditis, a lateral neck X-ray may be helpful. The X-ray may reveal a large volume of adenoid tissue obstructing the posterior choanae of the nasal cavity (Fig. **4**). Nasal endoscopy, a tool used by Otolaryngologists, gives valuable information in the evaluation of nasal issues. Although this is not used by primary care physicians, office nasal endoscopy allows inspection of the nasal cavity thoroughly at a patient's initial visit with a specialist. Nasal endoscopy can reveal polyp disease (Fig. **5**) Plain films of the sinuses is not helpful and does not give adequate detail of the anatomy to base clinical decisions, thus, it is rarely used.

Greater detail of the sinuses can be achieved with CT scans. Certainly in the pediatric population, CT scans should not be ordered for the routine diagnosis of sinusitis due to the concern of radiation exposure [7]. This type of imaging should be used if the diagnosis of sinusitis is in doubt, there are atypical features to the sinusitis or nasal problems, if there is concern for spread of the sinus infection to the orbits or intracranial, or if the potential for surgery exists. MRI is not often used for evaluation of the sinuses as it does not detail bony anatomy well. MRI can also be overly sensitive for inflammatory nasal disorders with a high false positive rate. The utility for MRI is for suspected intracranial complications.

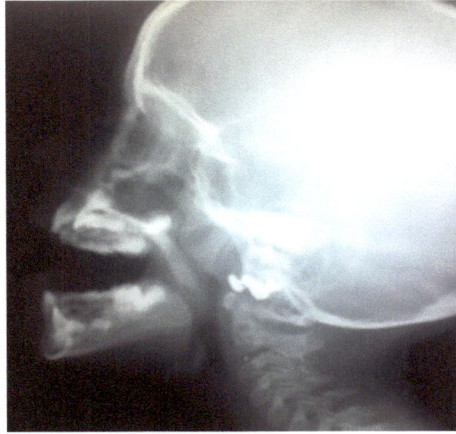

**Figure 4:** Enlarged Adenoid Obstructing the Posterior Choana.

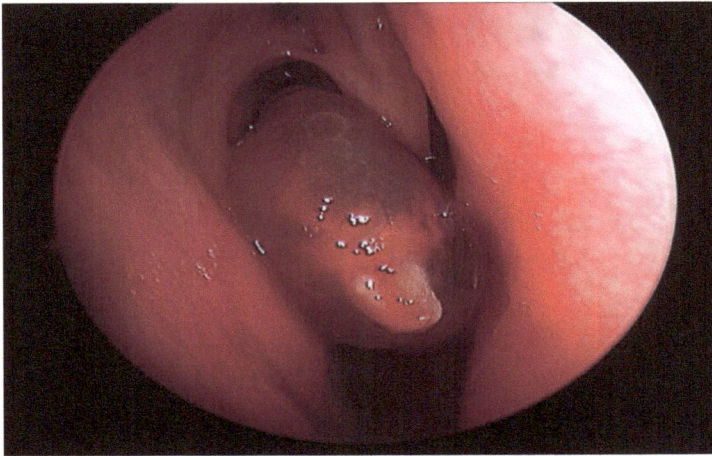

**Figure 5:** Nasal Polyp Visualized by Endoscopy.

For patients that have failed medical treatment for sinusitis or adenoiditis, surgery may be an option. Certainly adenoidectomy is a surgery that is performed often in children and has a good safety profile. For younger patients, the indications for adenoidectomy are nasal obstruction from adenoid tissue, recurrent sinusitis, and for chronic otitis media with effusion with concomitant nasal symptoms. An adenoidectomy is performed transorally and several methods exist for tissue removal. The tissue may be curetted out, cauterized, ablated or removed with a powered instrument called a microdebrider. This is typically based on surgeon preference. For patients with primary adenoid problems related to obstruction, the surgery is very successful. In patients with sinusitis, it may resolve symptoms but up to 50% of pediatric patients with sinusitis may continue to have symptoms [8].

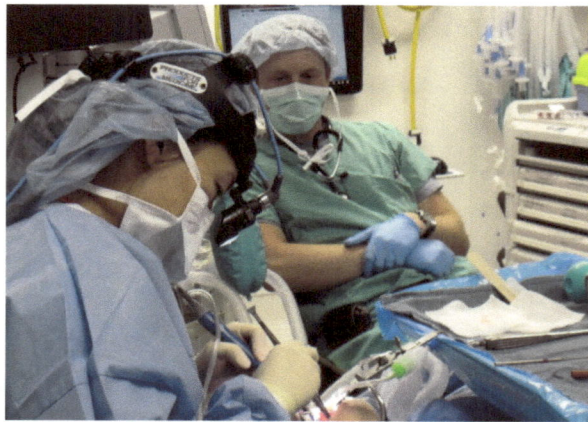

**Figure 6:** Otolaryngologist Performing Adenoidectomy.

Endoscopic sinus surgery is a procedure done frequently in adults with chronic sinus problems and not as often in children. The basic principle is to relieve obstruction at the natural openings of the sinuses to allow for more effective drainage (Fig. **6**). In addition, diseased tissue and polyps are removed. Topical antibiotics may be more effective in patients that have undergone endoscopic sinus surgery. Risks of endoscopic sinus surgery include orbital injury, intracranial injury, and scarring within the nasal cavity (Fig. **7**). An aggressive approach is not warranted in children and typically a limited sinus surgery is all that is necessary. Initially, there was concern for possible facial growth effects from sinus surgery but this has not been corroborated by evidence [9]. The trend towards less invasive surgery is manifested by the application of balloon technology to sinus surgery. The principle of this is to dilate the natural ostia of the sinuses with balloons, similar to angioplasty, to avoid tissue removal.

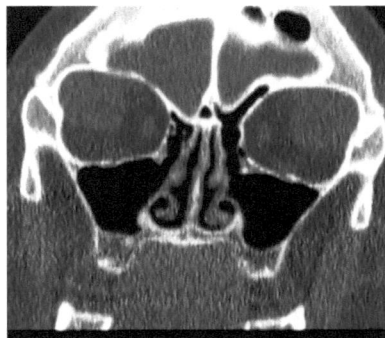

**Figure 7:** Nasal Cavity after Endoscopic Sinus Surgery.

The indications for endoscopic sinus surgery in children are controversial. With pediatric patients with chronic sinusitis, sinus surgery should not be performed until they have been thoroughly medically evaluated for comorbid conditions such as cystic fibrosis, ciliary dyskinesia, allergies, immunodeficiency and exposure to second-hand smoke. Following thorough evaluation, an appropriate course of antibiotics should be administered. A CT scan should be obtained following treatment if symptoms persist and,if the ostia appear obstructed and the sinuses have evidence of opacification, the child may be a candidate for formal sinus surgery.

## CONCLUSION

Sinusitis and adenoiditis are common entities encountered by primary care physicians and ENT specialists. With thorough diagnostic work-up, accurate diagnosis may be achieved and appropriate treatment can be initiated.

## ACKNOWLEDGEMENT

Declared none.

## CONFLICT OF INTEREST

The authors confirm that this chapter content has no conflict of interest.

## REFERENCES

[1]     Tan R, Spector S. Pediatric sinusitis. Curr Allergy Asthma Rep. 2007 Nov;7(6):421-6

[2]     Loehrl TA, Ferre RM, Toohill RJ, Smith TL Long-term asthma outcomes after endoscopic sinus surgery in aspirin triad patients.Am J Otolaryngol. 2006 May-Jun;27(3):154-60

[3]     Flook EP, Kumar BN.Is there evidence to link acid reflux with chronic sinusitis or any nasal symptoms. A review of the evidence. Rhinology. 2011 Mar; 49(1): 11-6

[4]     Rosbe KW, Jones DT, Rahbar R, Lahiri T, Auerbach AD Endoscopic sinus surgery in cystic fibrosis: do patients benefit from surgery? Int J Pediatr Otorhinolaryngol. 2001 Nov 1;61(2):113-9

[5]     Khalid AN, Hunt J, Perloff JR, Kennedy DW.The role of bone in chronic rhinosinusitis. Laryngoscope. 2002 Nov;112(11):1951-7

[6]     Suh JD, Ramakrishnan V, Palmer JN.Biofilms. Otolaryngol Clin North Am. 2010 Jun;43(3):521-30

[7]     Li X, Samei E, Segars WP.Patient-specific radiation dose and cancer risk estimation in CT: part II. Application to patients., Med Phys. 2011 Jan;38(1):408-19

[8]     Ramadan HH, Tiu J.Failures of adenoidectomy for chronic rhinosinusitis in children: for whom and when do they fail?.Laryngoscope. 2007 Jun;117(6):1080-3

[9]     Carpenter KM,Graham SM, Smith RJ.Facial skeletal growth after endoscopic sinus surgery in the piglet model. Am J Rhinol. 1997 May-Jun;11(3):211-7

*Send Orders of Reprints at reprints@benthamscience.net*
*Otolaryngology for the Pediatrician*, 2013, 95-108          95

# CHAPTER 6

# Approach to the Pediatric Patient with Sleep-Disordered Breathing

## Jessica J. Kepchar[1] and Scott E. Brietzke[2*]

*[1]Department of Otolaryngology, Walter Reed National Military Medical Center, Bethesda and [2]Department of Otolaryngology, Walter Reed National Military Medical Center, Bethesda, MD, USA*

**Abstract:** Sleep disordered breathing (SDB) is a commonly encountered medical problem in the pediatric patient population with varying ranges of severity including primary snoring, upper airway resistance syndrome and obstructive sleep apnea/hypopnea syndrome. While many clinicians are aware of certain risk factors that predispose children to obstructive sleep apnea syndrome, the prompt identification of all patients at risk for each of these syndromes is imperative. Clinicians currently use a combination of clinical indicators and polysomnographic data to diagnose children who may fall into the SDB spectrum. Without prompt diagnosis, a child be subject to multiple neurocognitive deficits, which may have been ameliorated by treatment. The appropriate treatment for obstructive sleep apnea hypopnea syndrome has traditionally been thought to be surgical, however, the ability to properly categorize children into the above spectrum of disorders will help a practitioner evaluate each patient individually and determine if surgery or other treatments are appropriate for a particular patient.

**Keywords:** Sleep disordered breathing, obstructive sleep apnea-hypopnea syndrome, upper airway resistance syndrome, snoring, polysomnogram, home sleep study, adenotonsillectomy.

## INTRODUCTION

Sleep disordered breathing (SDB) is a commonly encountered medical problem in the pediatric patient population with the primary symptom of nightly snoring afflicting approximately 10% of children [1-4]. It is this symptom that often brings the patient to the attention of the primary care provider and prompts an evaluation for obstructive sleep apnea. While sleep apnea is certainly a

---

*Address correspondence to Scott E. Brietzke: Department of Otolaryngology, Walter Reed National Military Medical Center, Bethesda, MD, USA; E-mail: Scott.brietzke@med.navy.mil

component of SDB, it actually is only one portion of the spectrum of entities associated with various degrees of upper airway obstruction in the pediatric patient. The varying severities of SDB span a spectrum from primary snoring (PS) to Upper Airway Resistance Syndrome (UARS) to Obstructive Sleep Apnea/Hypopnea Syndrome (OSAHS) (See Fig. **1**).

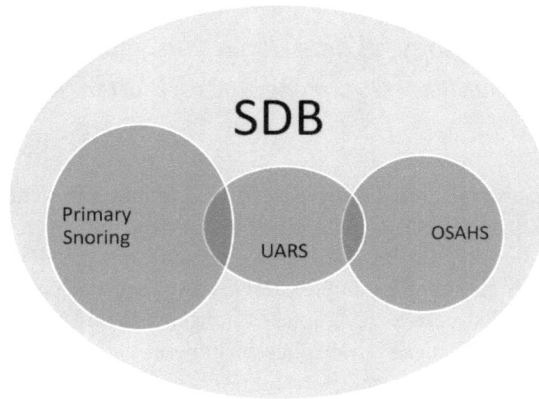

**Figure 1:** Ven Diagram illustrating the relationship between clinical entities within the realm of pediatric sleep disordered breathing. Note the size of the circles generally reflect relative prevalence of the clinical entitity.

Primary snoring is the presence of habitual snoring during the sleep cycle without findings commonly associated with obstruction such as pauses in breathing, gasping or frequent awakenings. Although PS is the mildest clinical entity on the SDB continuum, it is still associated with measurable negative clinical deficits. UARS encompasses those children who fall between primary snoring and frank obstruction and may be considered in the highly symptomatic child with partial airway obstruction resulting in episodes of heightened respiratory effort and resulting frequent arousals [1]. UARS is not associated with clearly identifiable apneas or hypopneas and is formally diagnosed with other measures in conjunction with polysomnography to include esophageal manometry, which readily identifies the pattern of increased respiratory effort that leads to arousals and sleep disruption. Finally, OSAHS represents the most severe category on the SDB continuum. The diagnosis of OSAHS is defined by the identification of apneas and/or hypopneas with associated abnormalities in gas exchange due to upper airway obstruction. It is essential that the provider who evaluates children with nighttime obstructive symptoms has a thorough knowledge of the disease process, its implications, and effective management strategies.

## Epidemiology

Sleep disordered breathing is a common pediatric problem. Nightly, habitual snoring affects approximately 10% of otherwise normal children [1-4]. While it obviously depends on the exact diagnostic criteria being used to define it, the estimated prevalence of OSAHS has been reported in the range of 0.7-3% of otherwise normal children [1,4-6]. Outside of the effects of obesity trends, these estimates appear to be relatively stable from one geographic area to another. Typically, the incidence of OSAHS will peak around the ages of 3-8 years old when tonsil and adenoid enlargement is greatest. There are certain risk factors and comorbidities that pose increased risk for development of SDB in the pediatric patient; however, the association of racial and socioeconomic factors with diagnosis of SDB has been explored. A recent systematic review found that children in racial and socioeconomic minorities may have greater prevalence and risk of developing SDB [2].

## Pathophysiology

The knowledge of the proper terminology and specific risk factors for SDB is important, however, it is a thorough understanding of the health concerns resulting from untreated SDB, particularly OSAHS that will encourage primary care practitioners to prioritize patients who present with concerning signs and symptoms. The pathophysiology of SDB is complex and not completely understood. It arises from the initial event of upper airway obstruction during sleep (See Fig. **2**).

This obstruction often occurs during periods of Rapid Eye movement (REM) sleep, where airway resistance is higher and probability of upper airway obstruction increases. This partial or complete obstruction of the airway is the initial event that sets off a cascade of events with far-reaching effects. The reason for the obstruction itself can be multi-factorial: pharyngeal and/or lingual tonsil enlargement, adenoid hypertrophy, and/or nasal inferior turbinate hypertrophy,

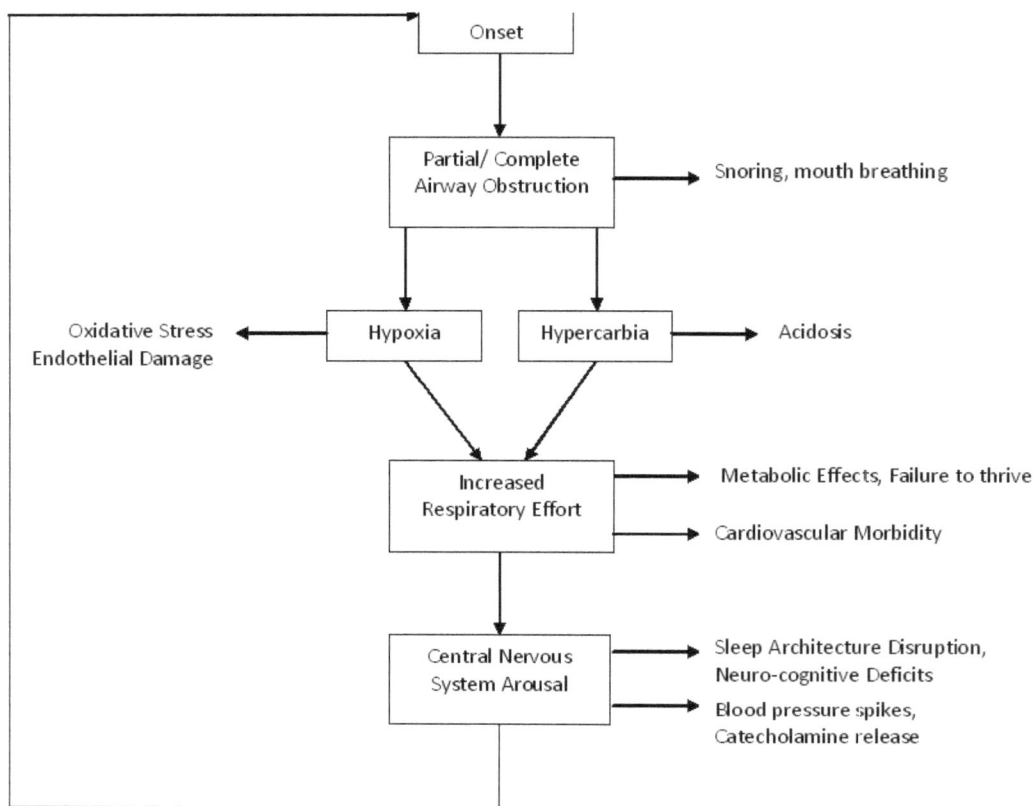

**Figure 2:** Simplified Schematic Diagram of the Pathophysiologic Mechanism of Sleep Disordered Breathing.

adipose tissue deposits within the walls of the pharynx, tongue enlargement or position (from the result of a syndrome such as Down's Syndrome or otherwise), or bony facial skeleton structure factors favoring increased airway collapsibility and development of obstructive events. Once the obstruction occurs, several resulting processes emerge with diverse consequences (See Fig. **2**). Within seconds of the obstruction, hypoxia (decreasing oxygen tension in the blood) and hypercarbia (increasing carbon dioxide tension) develop creating a metabolic turmoil to include acidosis and oxidative stress that can affect a multitude of organ systems. Subsequently, as the biochemical uproar from the obstruction quickly intensifies, respiratory effort is increased to relieve the obstruction and the muscle tone of the airway is increased to improve patency. In the majority of obstructive events, as the obstruction is relieved the event is terminated with an arousal from the sleep state within the central nervous system that is accompanied by a transient blood pressure spike, heart rate increase, and catecholamine release. Each of these events individually and collectively has its own cascade of effects that can produce a variety of problems and deficits in the pediatric patient. Clearly OSAHS produces the most severe sequelae for the patient. Yet to a lesser but still measurable degree, both PS and UARS also produce negative clinical consequences for the SDB patient particularly in the area of neurocognition.

The principle health concerns resulting from SDB include impaired neurocognitive functioning, failure to thrive, nocturnal enuresis and cardiovascular complications. Untreated SDB may increase the risk of developing deficits in multiple neurocognitive categories to include school performance, attention, intelligence and memory [7]. An improvement in cognitive function following adenotonsillectomy confirms this relationship.Traditionally, the children with severe SDB were of greater concern for physicians for developing cognitive deficits, however a recent study evaluating objective PSG data along with cognitive measures of intellectual ability, academic functioning and executive skills revealed that there was lower intellectual ability in patients with all ranges of SDB compared to control [7]. Theseresults help to confirm that each case of pediatric SDB should be considered separately and even mild cases on the clinical spectrum may require treatment depending on the associated presenting symptoms.

While pediatric obesity is more frequently documented in association with SDB, failure to thrive may also be associated with obstructive upper airway disorders. There is little published data to describe this relationship, however one study of 36 children with failure to thrive did note a 5.5% prevalence of PSG-diagnosed OSAHS, which indicates that patients with failure to thrive and appropriate symptoms should at least undergo an investigation for SDB [8].

A lesser known association between nocturnal enuresis and pediatric OSAHS has been reported in the literature. The exact cause for this relationship has not been definitely explained, however theories of insufficient sleep-time production of vasopressin, impaired urodynamics and increased levels of atrial natriuretic peptide have been postulated [9]. A retrospective study evaluating effectiveness of adenotonsillectomy on nocturnal enuresis was completed revealing that of the children evaluated for adenotonsillectomy, only the children who underwent surgery for SDB, not tonsillitis had associated findings of nocturnal enuresis [9]. Additionally, this study provided results that confirmed previous reports that nocturnal enuresis resolves or improves with adenotonsillectomy [9].

Perhaps the most imperative in terms of overall health and life expectancy of the patient are the cardiovascular consequences of SDB, particularly OSAHS. The acute autonomic alterations and endothelial dysfunction that results from recurring episodes of upper airway obstruction may lead to subsequent cardiovascular morbidity such as hypertension, pulmonary hypertension and impaired cerebral perfusion [6]. Certainly identifying SDB early in childhood and providing appropriate treatment may help to prevent translation of early vascular insult into chronic medical problems in later adolescence and adulthood.

## Evaluation

Armed with a concrete knowledge of the important health concerns revolving around SDB, a practitioner can better approach the history and physical exam in an effort to properly categorize children with concerns for upper airway obstruction. However, there are important limitations with the use of the clinical evaluation (*i.e.*, the history and physical exam) of which the provider must be aware when evaluating children for SDB. A recent systematic review of the literature has shown that the use of the history and physical alone are not reliable in all cases for diagnosing OSAHS when compared with the "gold standard" of overnight PSG [10]. The critical limitation to note is that while the positive predictive value (probability that SDB is present with the clinical evaluation is "positive") of the clinical evaluation is high, the negative predictive value is considerably lower (approximately 50%). Thus, combining this observation with the fact that the prevalence of SDB is very high in the snoring child, the provider can feel quite confident when ruling in the diagnosis of SDB based on the clinical exam, but ruling it out on this basis alone is problematic. It is **imperative** that the provider **does not** use the history and physical exam (especially tonsil size) alone to rule out SDB if they are suspicious of it. The negative predictive value of the clinical evaluation is simply not sufficient for this decision process and objective testing may be needed in these cases.

A good history of the SDB child should elicit several important points regarding the sleeping experience to include nightly snoring, witnessed apneas or pauses in breathing, choking or gasping, noisy or labored breathing, nocturnal enuresis and frequent arousals/restless sleep. However, it is **critical** to note that the absence of the parental report of these observations should **not** necessarily preclude a consideration of the diagnosis of SDB by the provider if they remain suspicious. Oftentimes, the parent(s) simply have not diligently monitored for these events or they occur later in the night/early morning hours (more typical of Rapid Eye Movement (REM) sleep when obstruction is more common) when a parent must sleep themselves and cannot observe the child. Additionally, the child's behavior, performance in school, developmental timeline and growth curve should be carefully documented and considered. The past medical history should also be explored to focus on the aforementioned risk factors, history of allergic disease and family history of SDB, although there is no know specific inheritance pattern for SDB.

An adequate physical exam should include an overall assessment of the patient's body habitus, oropharyngeal exam to include tonsillar evaluation and adenoid evaluation as indicated. Traditionally, the oropharyngeal exam with grading the tonsils on a 0-4+ scale has been used to predict which patients have more severe forms of SDB with increasing tonsil size being suggestive of more severe symptoms and therefore, a more severe diagnosis on the SDB continuum. However, this classical association is likely very **limited** and it is **essential** that the provider evaluating children with potential SDB is aware of this limitation. A recent systematic review has shown that the association between subjective pediatric tonsil size using this four point scale and objective data of SDB severity with polysomnography (PSG) is weak [11]. This translates to the reality that a patient with small tonsils should not be ruled out for SDB just because they have small tonsils, but rather objective testing with PSG should be pursued if clinical suspicion is present based on other clinical factors.

While adenotonsillar hypertrophy (ATH) certainly is a prime culprit when considering the etiology of pediatric SDB, a host of other factors increase the risk of development of SDB for certain pediatric patients and deserve attention from the provider. With the increased prevalence of obesity nationwide, the association of obesity with SDB is of great concern. It has been documented that both adenotonsillar hypertrophy as well as soft tissue hypertrophy secondary to obesity contribute to obstruction of the upper airway. However, it is unclear in what manner the distribution of adipose tissue within the head and neck actually contribute to the severity of SDB [3]. Moreover, the symptomatology of the obese child with SDB may be very different from that of the child with ATH. The obese child with SDB typically has a clinical presentation more similar to adults with SDB: somnolence, fatigue, and hypertension. Whereas, the typical child with SDB from ATH more commonly presents with the symptoms of hyperactivity and labile behavior issues.

Craniofacial abnormalities, particularly cleft anomalies (*e.g.*, Pierre Robin Sequence) and Down Syndrome (DS) are commonly associated with SDB. This observed association is due to problematic anatomic features such as macroglossia, facial hypoplasia and crowding of the oropharyngeal airway that favor obstruction [12]. Many syndromes may be associated with SDB, however the prevalence of DS in the general population makes it perhaps the most concerning syndromic risk factor for SDB. A reported incidence of OSAHS in the pediatric DS population ranges from 30-60%, and it may be difficult to diagnose based on history alone [13]. A prospective cohort study investigating whether DS children should be objectively tested determined that 69% of parents reported no sleep problems, however 54% of those patients had abnormal PSG results, whereas only 36% of DS patients had abnormal PSG results of the group in which parents reported sleep problems [13]. This information indicates the underestimation of symptoms by parents and the importance of objective testing prior to considering surgery in the pediatric DS patient. Another group of specialized patients who pose increased risk for SDB include those with diagnosis of neuromuscular diseases. While adenotonsillar hypertrophy may play a role in the obese child or even the child with craniofacial abnormalities, upper airway hypotonicity in the patient with neuromuscular afflictions such as Duchenne muscular dystrophy or cerebral palsy can play a larger role in the diagnosis of upper airway obstruction [1,14].

The polysomnogram (PSG) or sleep study has been the traditional "gold standard" for diagnosing OSAHS. In fact, the formal diagnostic criteria for diagnosis of each of the clinical entities of SDB are based on PSG criteria (See Tables **1, 2**).

**Table 1:** Common Polysomnography Terms related to Pediatric Sleep Disordered Breathing

| |
|---|
| **Obstructive Apnea:** cessation of airflow of greater than 90% for at least 2 respiratory cycles with continued respiratory effort. |
| **Obstructive Hypopnea:** reduction in airflow between 50-90% over two or more respiratory cycles with continued respiratory effort, accompanied by a 3% decrease in oxygen saturation and/or a Central Nervous System arousal. |
| **Respiratory Effort-Related Arousal (RERA):** increasing respiratory effort for 10 seconds or longer leading to an arousal from sleep that does not fulfill the criteria for a hypopnea or apnea, used for diagnosis of UARS (Note additional diagnostic techniques in conjunction with PSG such as esophageal manometry may be required for formal diagnosis). |
| **Central Apnea:** absence of airflow associated with absent respiratory effort. |
| **Mixed Apnea:** apnea with obstructive and central component with central component last >3 second. |
| **Apnea Hypopnea Index (AHI):** number of apneas and hypopneas divided by number of hours of sleep. |
| **Respiratory Disturbance Index (RDI)** – Often interchanged with AHI but actually includes the total number of apneas, hypopneas, and RERAs divided by the total hours of sleep. |

Currently, the criteria for an apnea (complete obstruction of the airway)is a 90% or greater cessation of airflow over two or more attempted respiratory cycles [15]. A hypopnea (partial airway obstruction) is defined as a greater than 50% reduction in airflow over two or more respiratory cycles, accompanied by a 3% decrease in oxygen saturation or an arousal [15]. It should be noted that these definitions do vary slightly between pediatric sleep laboratories; however, they do represent the generally accepted PSG parameters for diagnosing OSAHS.(See Table **2**)

**Table 2:** General Diagnostic Criteria for Pediatric Sleep Disordered Breathing.

| Diagnosis | Loud, Habitual Snoring | AHI | RERA Index | Comments |
|---|---|---|---|---|
| Primary Snoring | Yes | < 1.0 | < 10 | Loud snoring in the absence of other findings. Has been associated with neurocognitive deficits |
| Upper Airway Resistance Syndrome | Yes | < 1.0 | > 10 | Frequent arousals on sleep study in context of severe clinical sleepiness in absence of diagnostics criteria for OSAHS |
| Obstructive Sleep Apnea Hypopnea Syndrome | | | | Pediatric scoring generally reserved for patients 12 years and younger |
| Mild | Yes | ≥ 1-5 | Variable | |
| Moderate | Yes | 6-10 | Variable | |
| Severe | Yes | > 10 | Variable | |

AHI = Apnea Hypopnea Index
RERA = Respiratory Effort Related Arousal
OSAHS = Obstructive Sleep Apnea Hypopnea Syndrome

The total number of upper airway obstructions per hour to include apneas and hypopneas is defined as the apnea hypopnea index (AHI) and is considered statistically abnormal in the pediatric patient when it exceeds an average of one event per hour. However, the precise objective definitions of SDB that lead to persistent negative clinical implications and that warrant directed treatment have not been clearly defined.

Although PSG is attractive as it provides objective data that are somewhat correlated to patient operative risk and outcomes, it is not practical in many cases. It is expensive (multiple $1000s in most areas) and labs that conduct pediatric studies of suitable quality are not available in many parts of the country. Also, it is burdensome to the family and patient to schedule the study, gain insurance approval if necessary, complete the study, and then return to the referring provider with a completed study report. This cumbersome process often results in delays in care that last for weeks to months. Thus, having clear and focused clinical criteria on when to employ this limited resource would seem appropriate. Unfortunately, consensus on this topic has been elusive with many diverse groups involved in the clinical area of pediatric SDB to include pediatricians, otolaryngologists, sleep medicine experts, pediatric pulmonologists, and pediatric neurologists. Recently, the American Academy of Otolaryngology produced a clinical practice guideline on the use of pediatric PSG prior to tonsillectomy [6]. The recommendations for obtaining PSG included patients with higher than average risk for surgery (Craniofacial syndromes, Obesity, neuromuscular disorders, *etc.*) and for cases where the clinical severity of SDB does not correlate with the physical exam, *i.e.,* areas of diagnostic uncertainty. This would seem to be a reasonable place to start. However, little has been discussed about the potentially much more beneficial role for PSG in assessing patients after treatment to detect and quantify residual SDB. More study in this area is certainly warranted and would seem to be of high priority to appropriately guide the care of large numbers of pediatric patients with SDB. The use of less expensive, more convenient home sleep testing technology in the evaluation of the pediatric SDB patient would seem to be an inviting solution to this dilemma. Unfortunately, this technology is only in the initial stages of development and has not been rigorously evaluated or widely embraced. Yet, it could ultimately prove to be a useful tool to provide cost effective, additional objective data to assist with diagnosis of SDB and the assessment of SDB treatment effectiveness.

## Treatment

Because of the primacy of adenotonsillar hypertrophy as the assumed etiology of the majority of pediatric SDB, removal of the tonsils and adenoids (T/A) has been considered by most to be the first step in uncomplicated pediatric SDB management. And given the overall excellent safety record of T/A and its high success rate (70-80% cure in the uncomplicated, non-obese patient), it likely should remain as the first line therapy for the majority of uncomplicated patients with pediatric OSAHS [15]. However, the appropriate therapy for pediatric PS and UARS remains less clear. Although the morbidity of PS and UARS are certainly less than OSAHS they have been clearly demonstrated to have negative clinical implications and further study of the appropriate treatment for these common problems is undoubtedly indicated.

Pediatric T/A is a commonly performed procedure with an excellent safety record. Over 500,000 pediatric tonsillectomies are performed in the US alone and this number seems to be climbing [2]. Serious complications from tonsillectomy are rare and include post-operative hemorrhage (1-3% of patients) or anesthesia complications (<1%). Death from tonsillectomy is exceedingly rare and although data of this type are hard to compile, it is clearly well less than 1%. T/A has a well-known morbidity in terms of throat pain and dietary alteration with most children (and thus their caregivers also) requiring 7-10 days to fully recover from surgery. Alternative methods of tonsillectomy to include electrocautery, radiofrequency ablation, microdebrider removal, and even partial tonsillectomy techniques are areas of intense investigation in an attempt to reduce post-operative pain. Consensus on the ideal method of surgery has not been established and remains elusive with many opinions but insufficient comparative data. The majority of T/A cases are performed on a same day basis with overnight observation generally occurring in higher risk patients such as children less than 2 years of age, Down syndrome patients, extremely obese patients, and patients with neuromuscular disorders or bleeding dyscrasias. Probably the greatest limitation of T/A is its imperfect success rate (particularly in obese patients) in combination with the frequency in which it is performed. Although the success rate of T/A in uncomplicated patients is high, it is not 100%. Thus, given the reality that over 500,000 T/As are performed each year, the possibility of residual SDB after surgery is a definite issue that must appropriately addressed. Assessing and evaluating appropriate treatment for residual SDB after T/A is perhaps the **greatest** priority in pediatric SDB research as this is likely a very common but under-diagnosed problem with unknown consequences.

Beyond T/A, many treatments for pediatric SDB have been described. In the obese pediatric patient, medical management may encompass weight loss or continuous positive airway pressure (CPAP). Weight loss may be considered a reasonable first-line therapy for the obese patient, however, there is little prospective data to support this approach [3]. Likewise, CPAP, while the first-line therapy for adult OSA, actually has insufficient data to support long-term use in the pediatric patient [3]. One recent study of 29 children, of which two thirds were documented as obese, revealed efficacy for both CPAP and bilevel pressure (BiPAP), however, treatment with both forms were associated with a high dropout rate due to the commonly accepted nuances of using this type of therapy such as equipment issues, adverse nasal symptoms and skin complaints from use of the mask [17]. This is of course homologous to the experience with CPAP in adult SDB patients where CPAP effectiveness is high but long-term compliance is suboptimal. Medical therapy with nasal steroids and leukotriene inhibitors has also shown to be moderately effective in objectively reducing OSAHS [18]. Yet, determining the end point for this therapy can be troublesome and has not been adequately described. Regardless of the current limitations of therapies beyond T/A, the need to explore and develop current therapies further as well as cultivate additional therapies is critical as the number of pediatric patients with residual OSAHS after T/A is increasing, particularly as pediatric obesity continues to rise.

## Outcomes/Future Directions

Pediatric SDB is an increasingly common problem with imperfect solutions. Evaluation of the SDB patient can be difficult due to limitations in the history and physical exam being limited, cumbersome objective testing. Home sleep testing is being developed may be a potential solution for this problem. Surgery is currently a mainstay of first line management as tonsillectomy and adenoidectomy is a safe and effective (although imperfect) treatment in the uncomplicated patient. However, the sheer volume of SDB patients along with the rise of obesity has resulted in increasing numbers of patients that have residual SDB after surgery. Development of criteria for patients with residual disease that would benefit from further treatment and the development of effective additional treatments for SDB (both medical and surgical) should be a pediatric public health priority.

## ACKNOWLEDGEMENT

Declared none.

## CONFLICT OF INTEREST

The authors confirm that this chapter content has no conflict of interest.

## DISCLOSURE

Please note the views herein are the private views of the authors and do not reflect the official views of the Department of Defense or the Department of the Army.

## REFERENCES

[1]     1 Sterni L and Tunkel D. "Obstructive Sleep Apnea Syndrome." *Cummings Otolaryngology Head and Neck Surgery.* Philadelphia: Elsevier 2010.

[2]     Boss E, Smith D, Ishman S. Racial/ethnic and socioeconomic disparities in the diagnosis and treatment of sleep-disordered breathing in children. *Int Jour Ped Oto* 2011; 75: 299-307.

[3]     Verhulst SL, Van Gaal L, *et al.* The prevalence, anatomical correlates and treatment of sleep-disordered breathing in obese children and adolescents. *Sleep Medicine Reviews* 2008; 12: 339-346.

[4]     Brietzke SE, Katz ES, Roberson DW. Pulse transit time as a screening test for pediatric sleep-related breathing disorders. *Arch Otolaryngol Head Neck Surg* 2007; 133(10): 980-984.

[5]     Brietzke SE, Gallagher D. The effectiveness of tonsillectomy and adenoidectomy in the treatment of pediatric obstructive sleep apnea/hypopnea syndrome: A meta-analysis. *Otolaryngol Head Neck Surg* 2006; 134: 979-984.

[6]     Kheirandish-Gozal L, Bhattacharjee R, Gozal D. Autonomic alterations and endothelial dysfunction in pediatric obstructive sleep apnea. *Sleep Medicine* 2010; 11: 714-720.

[7]     Bourke R, Anderson V, *et al.* Cognitive and academic functions are impaired in children with all severities of sleep-disordered breathing. *Sleep Medicine* 2011; 12: 489-496.

[8]     Stone RS, Spiegel JH. Prevalence of obstructive sleep disturbance in children with failure to thrive. *J Otolaryngol Head Neck Surg* 2009; 38(5): 573-9.

[9]     Basha S, Bialowas C, *et al.* Effectiveness of adenotonsillectomy in the resolution of nocturnal enuresis secondary to obstructive sleep apnea. *Laryngoscope* 2005;115: 1101-1103.

[10]    Brietzke S, Katz E, Roberson D. Can history and physical examination reliably diagnose pediatric obstructive sleep apnea/hypopnea syndrome? A systematic review of the literature. *Otolaryngol Head Neck Surg* 2004; 131:827-32.

[11]    Nolan J, Brietzke S. Systematic review of pediatric tonsil size and polysomnogram-measures obstructive sleep apnea severity. *Otolaryngol Head Neck Surg* 2011; 144(6): 844-50.

[12]    Lam D, Jensen C, *et al.* Pediatric sleep apnea and craniofacial anomalies: A population-based case-control study. *Laryngoscopy* 2010; 120: 2098-2105.

[13]    Shott S, Amin R, el al. Obstructive Sleep Apnea: Should all children with Down syndrome be tested? *Arch Otolaryngol Head Neck Surg* 2006; 132: 432-436.

[14]    Katz S. Assessment of sleep-disordered breathing in pediatric neuromuscular diseases. *Pediatrics* 2009; 123: S222-S224.

[15]    Uliel S, Tauman R, Greenfeld M, Sivan Y. Normal polysomnographic respiratory values in children and adolescents. *Chest* 2004; 125: 872-878.

[16]    Roland P, Rosenfeld R, Brooks L, *et al.* Clinical practice guideline: polysomnography for sleep-disordered breathing prior to tonsillectomy for children. *Otolaryngol Head Neck Surg* 2011; S1-S12.

[17]    Marcus CL, Rosen G, Davidson S, *et al.* Adherence to and effectiveness of positive airway pressure therapy in children with obstructive sleep apnea. *Pediatrics* 2006; 117: e442-e451.

[18]    Gozal D, Kheirandish L. Sleep apnea in children-treatment considerations. *Paediatric Resp Reviews* 2006; 7S:S58-S61.

*Send Orders of Reprints at reprints@benthamscience.net*

# CHAPTER 7

## Pediatric Otolaryngology Emergencies

### Jonathan R. Mark and Cristina M. Baldssari[*]

*Eastern Virginia Medical School, Department of Otolaryngology- Head and Neck Surgery, Norfolk, Virginia, USA*

**Abstract:** Clinicians must be familiar with the evaluation and treatment of common pediatric otolaryngology emergencies such as airway obstruction, head and neck trauma, caustic ingestion, airway and esophageal foreign bodies, and epistaxis. Pediatric otolaryngology emergencies frequently involve the airway. Etiologies for airway obstruction in children are diverse and include disease processes like croup, bacterial tracheitis, and angioedema. The majority of children with foreign body aspiration do not present with acute airway compromise. These patients often have non-specific symptoms such as chronic cough. Thus, the provider must have a high index of suspicion to make the diagnosis of an airway foreign body. While laryngeal trauma in children is rare, findings such as neck crepitus and stridor warrant further evaluation to rule out pathology such as laryngeal fracture. The majority of cases of pediatric epistaxis can be managed conservatively with topical decongestants and chemical cautery of the anterior septum.

**Keywords:** Airway obstruction, stridor, croup, epiglottitis, angioedema, bacterial tracheitis, laryngeal trauma, oropharyngeal trauma, traumatic tympanic membrane perforation, caustic ingestion, inhalation injury, airway foreign body, esophageal foreign body, ear foreign body, nasal foreign body, epistaxis.

## INTRODUCTION

Many children that present for otolaryngology evaluation have non-urgent conditions that can be managed on an outpatient basis. However, there are certain otolaryngology emergencies that require more immediate intervention. This chapter focuses on the evaluation and management of common pediatric otolaryngology emergencies including airway obstruction, head and neck trauma, caustic ingestion, airway and esophageal foreign bodies, and epistaxis.

---

*Address correspondence to Cristina Baldassari: Eastern Virginia Medical School, Department of Otolaryngology- Head and Neck Surgery, Norfolk, Virginia, USA; E-mail: Cristina.Baldassari@chkd.org

## AIRWAY OBSTRUCTION

Pediatric otolaryngology emergencies frequently involve the airway. Algorithms in pediatric life support exist with evidence-based guidelines for a systematic approach to assessment and management of the airway [1]. Need for emergent surgical airway is rare in pediatrics. However, trachetomy may be utilized if other attempts at securing the airway have failed. Cricothyroidotomy is not commonly performed in children due to difficulty identifying surgical landmarks and the small caliber of the airway.

Airway obstruction in children can lead to cardiorespiratory failure. The etiologies of acute airway obstruction in pediatric patients are numerous. Examples are listed in (Table 1) and will be further discussed in subsequent paragraphs. The clinician must recognize signs of airway obstruction and intervene to prevent further deterioration of the patient's clinical status. Common findings associated with impending airway obstruction are increased respiratory rate, stridor, chest retractions, peri-oral cyanosis, and oxygen desaturation. Other signs of respiratory failure are nasal alar flaring, lethargy, and hypercarbia. In addition to obtaining vital signs and performing a brief clinical assessment, other tests such as lateral neck and chest X-rays, blood gas, and flexible fiberoptic laryngoscopy may also be useful in evaluating a child with airway obstruction. In scenarios involving acute airway obstruction, the clinician should avoid any stimulation of the patient that might hasten impending respiratory failure. Interventions for pediatric airway obstruction include oxygen supplementation, intravenous steroids, racemic epinephrine treatments, endotracheal intubation, and placement of a surgical airway. In children with acute obstruction and respiratory failure, the airway is best managed in a controlled setting, such as the operating room, where direct laryngoscopy and bronchoscopy can be performed with equipment for tracheostomy at the ready.

**Table 1:** Causes of Airway Obstruction in Pediatric Patients.

| Nose/Nasopharynx |
| --- |
| Choanal atresia/stenosis |
| Nasolacrimal Duct Cyst |
| Midline nasal masses |

*Table 1: contd...*

| |
|---|
| Rhinitis |
| Adenoid hypertrophy |
| Trauma |
| **Oropharynx and Hypopharynx** |
| Micrognathia |
| Macroglossia |
| Tonsillar hypertrophy |
| Vallecular cyst |
| Deep neck space infection |
| Foreign body |
| **Supraglottis** |
| Laryngomalacia |
| Laryngeal cyst/laryngocele |
| Supraglottitis/Epiglottitis |
| Angioedema |
| Lymphatic malformation |
| **Glottis** |
| Laryngeal web |
| Laryngeal cleft |
| Vocal cord paralysis |
| Foreign body |
| Trauma |
| Papilloma |
| Paradoxical vocal fold movement |
| **Subglottis** |
| Subglottic stenosis |
| Subglottic cyst |
| Croup |
| Hemangioma |
| **Tracheobronchial** |
| Tracheomalacia |
| Tracheal web |
| Bacterial tracheitis |
| Complete tracheal rings |
| Foreign body |

## SYMPTOMS OF AIRWAY OBSTRUCTION

### Stridor

Stridor is not a disease, rather it is a clinical symptom of airway obstruction. Stridor is a harsh, high-pitched sound produced by turbulent airflow through an obstructed airway [2]. Stridor can be associated with diseases that range from mild to life-threatening in severity. The clinician must distinguish which children presenting with stridor are at risk for acute airway obstruction and respiratory failure and initiate appropriate treatment strategies.

The type of stridor can aid the clinician in determining the level of airway obstruction. High pitched inspiratory stridor is often associated with supraglottic pathology. Obstruction at the glottis and subglottis often produces biphasic stridor which occurs during both inspiration and expiration. Stridor must be distinguished from both wheezing, an expiratory whistle caused by collapse of the bronchi during expiration, and stertor, a low-pitched inspiratory sound produced by nasal obstruction [2]. Acute, progressive stridor associated with signs of impending airway obstruction such as retractions and cyanosis requires emergent evaluation and management as detailed above.

## ETIOLOGIES OF AIRWAY OBSTRUCTION

Many of the common causes of acute airway obstruction in children are inflammatory in nature. Disease processes such as croup, deep neck space infections, epiglottitis, angioedema, and bacterial tracheitis are considered otolaryngology emergencies when associated with airway compromise.

### Croup

Croup or acute laryngotracheobronchitis is characterized by barking cough and inspiratory or biphasic stridor secondary to subglottic inflammation. Croup is caused by the parainfluenza virus and usually affects children six months to five years of age. Treatment is tailored to symptom severity and entails humidified air, supplemental oxygen, racemic epinephrine, and steroids. Intubation is rarely necessary, but is utilized in children with respiratory failure.

## Deep Space Neck Infections

Common deep neck space infections in children include parapharyngeal, retropharyngeal, and peri-tonsillar cellulitis and abscess. Fascial planes in the deep neck spaces have pathways of communication that can extend locally or distantly, in some instances to the mediastinum. This allows for complications including airway compression, thrombosis of the great vessels, Horner syndrome, and mediastinitis. The majority of children with deep neck space infections do not present in extremis. However, the presence of certain clinical findings including dyspnea, stridor, drooling, lethargy, and trismus should alert the clinician of a potentially complicated case. In a stable patient, imaging studies such as computed tomography (CT) may be utilized to determine the extent of disease and aid in surgical planning. Treatment of deep neck space infections should be tailored to the patient based on the acuity and severity of the clinical picture. Securing the airway in a patient with respiratory distress is the first priority. Oral intubation in a patient with a deep neck space infection may be difficult. Anatomic distortion, potential for abscess rupture leading to aspiration, and trismus, present a challenge even for the experienced practitioner.

## Epiglottitis

Epiglottitis is an acute onset of inflammation and edema in the supraglottis. Prior to the Haemophilus influenzae type b (Hib) vaccine, this disease was a common cause of airway obstruction in children. The incidence of acute epiglottitis in the pediatric population has dramatically declined in the last several decades. In a study from Denmark, the annual incidence of epiglottitis declined from 4.9 cases per 100, 000 persons to 0.02 cases per 100 000 following the introduction of the Hib vaccine [3].

Common presenting signs and symptoms of epiglottitis include stridor, sore throat, fever, drooling, and dysphagia. The patient may present in the sniffing position with the body leaning forward and the head and nose pointed upward in an attempt to maintain a patent airway. This should alert the clinician to the possibility of impending respiratory failure. In some cases it may be difficult to differentiate epiglottitis from croup. There are several clinical features that help to distinguish between these two disease processes (Table **2**). For example, Tibballs *et al.* studied the early clinical presentation of children with epiglottitis and croup. The authors noted that the occurrence of coughing in the absence of drooling was characteristic of croup, while drooling in the absence of coughing was more characteristic of epiglottitis [4].

**Table 2:** Croup *vs.* Epiglottitis.

|  | CROUP | EPIGLOTTITIS |
|---|---|---|
| **Age at presentation** | 3 months to 3 years | 2 to 7 years |
| **X-ray findings** | subglottic narrowing (steeple-sign) | enlarged epiglottis (thumb-print sign) |
| **Chronology** | onset hours to days | onset hours |
| **General** | nontoxic | toxic |
| **Cough** | barking | absent |
| **Drooling** | absent | present |

Epiglottitis is a clinical diagnosis. If epiglottis is suspected, the provider should avoid agitating the child. Non-essential manipulation of the patient such as examination of the oral cavity with a tongue blade should be avoided. Quickly securing the airway is paramount in a child with suspected epiglottitis. This is best done in a controlled setting in the operating room. A direct laryngoscopy is performed with a tracheostomy set-up ready. Cultures are obtained from the larynx and an endotracheal tube is placed. Broad-spectrum antibiotics are started.

**Angioedema**

Angioedema is rapid onset (minutes to hours) swelling of mucous membranes, submucosal tissues, and dermis due to an increase of local vascular permeability. Angioedema usually involves the face, upper airway, and extremities. A common cause of angioedema is medications including angiotension converting enzyme (ACE) inhibitors. There is also a hereditary form of angioedema which is an autosomal dominant disease characterized by decreased functional C1-esterase inhibitor.

Angioedema involving the face, oral cavity, and pharynx can become a critical problem due to airway obstruction. During clinical evaluation, symptoms such as voice changes, dysphagia, and stridor may be a sign of upper airway involvement and thus warrant further investigation. In such patients, flexible fiberoptic laryngoscopy should be performed to assess for airway patency. If there is evidence of significant pharyngeal or laryngeal involvement, early airway intervention is warranted as rapid clinical deterioration can occur in patients with angioedema. Awake fiberoptic intubation is preferred over conventional direct laryngoscopy intubation in patients with swelling of the tounge, palate, and supraglottis. Medical therapies such as histamine blockers and corticosteroids can be helpful in reducing swelling in mast cell mediated disease. Hereditary angioedema may be treated with fresh frozen plasma (FFP) or ecallantide (a kallikrein inhibitor that inhibits the conversion of high molecular weight kininogen to bradykinin).

## Bacterial Tracheitis

Bacterial tracheitis is an acute, potentially life-threatening infection of the airway resulting in edema, sloughing of the tracheal epithelial lining, and accumulation of mucopurulent debris in the tracheal lumen. While the exact etiology of bacterial tracheitis is unknown, the disease process may represent a bacterial superinfection of croup. Children between the ages of 2 and 8 are most commonly affected. Younger children are often toxic on presentation with high fevers, lethargy, stridor, and a croup-like cough. Typically the symptoms do not respond to conventional therapies like inhaled racemic epinephrine. The presentation of bacterial tracheitis in older children may be more indolent and is characterized by low grade fevers, subjective dyspnea, and hoarseness [5]. In affected children, the lateral neck X-ray may show sloughing of the tracheal epithelium. Flexible fiberoptic laryngoscopy is another useful tool in the evaluation of a child with potential bacterial tracheitis. Crusting and purulence noted in the subglottis on flexible scope suggests the diagnosis.

The gold standard for the diagnosis of bacterial tracheitis is direct laryngoscopy and bronchoscopy performed in the operating room. Endoscopy is both diagnostic and therapeutic allowing the surgeon to remove the tracheal debris and send tracheal aspirates for culture. Depending on the amount of airway edema, children may require intubation for 24 to 48 hours. Management also includes initiating broad spectrum antibiotic therapy. *Staphylococcus aureus* is the most commonly implicated bacterial organism in bacterial tracheitis, followed by *Streptococcus pneumoniae*, *Haemophilus influenzae*, *Streptococcus pyogenes*, and *Pseudomonas* [6]. In a review by Huang, cases of pseudomonas tracheitis tended to have a more severe course [7]. Proactive management with endoscopy and antibiotic therapy decreased the rate of complications and the need for intubation and tracheotomy in patients with bacterial tracheitis [5].

## TRAUMA

### Laryngeal Trauma

Laryngeal trauma in children is rare due to certain inherent characteristics of the pediatric larynx such as pliable cartilage, high position in the neck, and shielding by the mandible. When injury does occur, the small size of the larynx and the weakness of the membranes may lead to severe consequences [8]. Mechanisms of injury include penetrating and blunt trauma. Falls onto sharp objects or edges and clothes line-type injuries from motorized vehicles are examples of such traumas.

The clinician must have a high index of suspicion to identify and appropriately manage laryngeal trauma in children. Signs of laryngeal trauma include anterior neck ecchymosis, flattening of the thyroid cartilage contour, subcutaneous emphysema (crepitus), stridor, and hoarseness. There are numerous different types of pathology that can result from laryngeal trauma including mucosal lacerations and hematomas, laryngeal fractures, vocal cord paralysis, arytenoid dislocation, and cricotracheal separation. In a patient with suspected laryngeal trauma, endotracheal intubation should be avoided as distortion of laryngeal anatomy may make visualization difficult. Furthermore, intubation may increase the separation of the cricoid and first tracheal ring in cases of cricotracheal separation. In an emergent situation in which the airway is tenuous, a tracheotomy under local anesthesia may be performed. In a patient with a stable airway and no respiratory distress, diagnostic tests such as flexible fiberoptic laryngoscopy and computed tomography with fine cuts through the larynx may provide the clinician with additional information about the extent of laryngeal trauma.

### Oropharyngeal Trauma

Oropharyngeal trauma may occur when a child falls with an object in his/her mouth. Common items that are implicated in oropharyngeal trauma in children are sticks, pencils, utensils, and toothbrushes. Palatal contusions, lacerations, and puncture wounds are frequently observed in cases of oropharyngeal trauma. Complications such as exsanguination and rapidly expanding hematoma due to direct disruption of the carotid artery are very rare. However, blunt injuries to the oropharynx in the area of the palate can result in intimal disruption of the carotid artery which can lead to thrombosis, dissection, and/or cerebral ischemia [9]. Radiographic screening for vascular injury in children presenting after oroparhyngeal trauma remains controversial, but are indicated in instances of focal neurological signs and symptoms [10]. Proposed studies include CTA, arteriography, ultrasound, and MRA. Extensive lacerations may require repair in the operating room. Children with oropharyngeal trauma are frequently admitted for overnight observation.

## Traumatic Tympanic Membrane Perforation

Traumatic tympanic membrane perforations may occur as a result of air/water pressure or penetrating objects such as Q-tips. Common symptoms include pain, aural fullness, and bloody otorrhea. Blood and debris should be carefully suctioned out of the ear canal to allow for an accurate assessment of the perforation size and location. Irrigation is avoided. Additional complications such as ossicular chain discontinuity, sensorineural hearing loss, and a perilymph fistula may occur in the setting of traumatic tympanic membrane perforation. Such children may present with vertigo, tinnitus, and hearing loss and require an emergent referral to an otolaryngologist for audiologic and clinical assessment. Most small perforations resolve spontaneously. Patients are advised to avoid letting water enter the ear. Perforations that fail to heal after weeks to months may require surgical repair [11].

## CAUSTIC INGESTION AND INHALATION INJURY

Oral, pharyngeal, laryngeal, or esophageal injuries may occur as a result of caustic ingestion. Unlike in adults, the majority of cases of caustic ingestion in children are accidental with the highest incidence occurring in children less than five years of age. When possible, it is important to ascertain the identity of the substance ingested by the child as the type and severity of the injury is often related to the pH of substance. Alkaline ingestions, such as drain cleaners, cause tissue injury by liquefactive necrosis. Cell death occurs from emulsification and disruption of cellular membranes which allows diffusion of corrosive material into deeper layers. Acid ingestions, such as rust removal agents, cause tissue injury by coagulation necrosis, which often results in the formation of an eschar that protects the underlying tissue from further damage. Thus, injuries sustained from ingestion of alkali substances are frequently more severe than those caused by ingestion of acidic substances. Bleach, a relatively neutral substance, may induce local tissue edema when ingested but does not typically cause extensive necrosis.

Children that have ingested a caustic material may present with drooling, odynophagia, and burns to their face and mouth. Initial management should include limiting exposure to the concentrated substance through irrigating contact sites. Providers should avoid inducing emesis with agents such as charcoal as regurgitation of the caustic agent can cause further injury to the esophagus and pharynx. Fluid resuscitation should be initiated on presentation. In a patient with a stable airway, further testing such as a metabolic panel to assess for any electrolyte imbalances and a chest X-ray to assess for mediastinitis may be warranted. Barium swallow is not indicated in the acute evaluation of child with caustic ingestion.

Endoscopic evaluation is the gold standard for determining the extent of esophageal injury in a patient with caustic ingestion. Endoscopy, whether it be flexible or rigid, allows the clinician to determine the depth of injury to the esophageal mucosa. This is important for prognosis and management. Grade 1 injuries, which are the least severe, are characterized by mucosal erythema while grade 4 injuries involve perforation of the esophageal wall (Table **3**). Grade 1 and 2 injuries are typically managed by observation and supportive care. Grade 3 injuries necessitate nasogastric tube placement under direct visualization. Children with grade 4 injuries are at increased risk for complications like mediastinitis and require operative open operative repair of the esophagus. The use of antibiotics and steroids in the setting of caustic ingestion are controversial. Late complications of caustic ingestion include stricture formation and esophageal cancer. Children with grade 2 and 3 injuries require either a repeat endoscopy or a barium swallow 3 weeks after the initial ingestion to assess for strictures.

**Table 3:** Grades of Esophageal Injury in Caustic Ingestion.

| Esophageal Injury | Depth | Endoscopic Findings | Treatment |
|---|---|---|---|
| Grade I | superficial mucosal injury | mucosal hyperemia and edema | observation and supportive care |
| Grade II | partial thickness injury | mucosal sloughing with superficial and deep ulcers, linear or patchy | observation and supportive care with repeat endoscopy or barium swallow 3 weeks after initial ingestion to assess for strictures |
| Grade III | circumferential injury with sloughing of the mucosa | mucosal sloughing with superficial ulcers and deep ulcers, circumferential | nasogastric tube placement under direct visualization with repeat endoscopy or barium swallow 3 weeks after initial ingestion to assess for strictures |
| Grade IV | perforation of the esophageal wall | perforation of the esophageal wall | operative repair of the esophagus |

## FOREIGN BODIES

### Airway Foreign Body

Aspirated foreign bodies may obstruct the airway at the level of the larynx, trachea, or bronchi. Foreign body aspiration accounts for 7% of lethal accidents in children 1 to 3 years of age. In the United States, 80% of aspirated materials are vegetable matter with peanuts being the most common. Children that aspirate rubber balloons have a higher risk of asphyxiation than those aspirating other objects [12].

Recognition of complete *vs.* partial airway obstruction is essential for first responders. A coughing or gagging child does not have complete airway obstruction. Attempts to dislodge the foreign body by interventions such as inverting the child are not recommended as they have the potential to turn partial airway obstruction into complete obstruction. A child whose airway is completely obstructed by a foreign body will be unable to speak or cough. This is an emergent situation. Attempts should be made to dislodge the foreign body by back blows and chest thrusts in children less than 1 year of age and by gentle abdominal thrusts in older children.

The majority of children with foreign body aspiration do not present in acute distress. The presentation of a child with an airway foreign body can be nonspecific. Thus, the provider must have a high index of suspicion to make the diagnosis of foreign body aspiration. Obtaining an accurate history is essential in the evaluation. A history of a witnessed aspiration or choking episode has a higher sensitivity than either physical exam or chest X-ray in the diagnosis of foreign body aspiration [13]. A young child that presents after a choking or gagging episode should be considered to have a foreign body until proven otherwise even in the absence of any physical exam or radiologic abnormalities. The presentation of foreign body aspiration can also be delayed. The provider should consider foreign body aspiration in children with recurrent pneumonias of unknown etiology and in those presenting with acute onset wheezing and asthma that were previously healthy. Physical exam findings in a patient with an airway foreign body may include stridor, tachypnea, diminished breath sounds, and wheezing. However, many children with foreign body aspiration have a normal physical exam.

Imaging studies may be useful in the evaluation of a child with suspected foreign body aspiration. A chest X-ray, ideally an expiratory view, should be obtained. Expiratory chest X-ray findings that suggest foreign body aspiration include lung hyperinflation on the affected side and mediastinal shift to the opposite side. Young children may have difficulty cooperating with inspiration and expiration during imaging. In such children, a lateral decubitus film should be obtained. A bronchial foreign body should be suspected if the dependent lung fails to deflate on a lateral decubitus film. A normal chest X-ray does not rule out foreign body aspiration. Airway fluoroscopy and computed tomography (CT) scan of the chest are other imaging modalities that have been utilized in children presenting with possible airway foreign body. However, these studies are not indicated for routine use in the evaluation of a child with suspected foreign body aspiration.

Direct laryngoscopy with rigid bronchoscopy is both diagnostic and therapeutic for foreign body aspiration. The procedure should be performed in a controlled setting in the operating room by a team of providers, including nurses, anesthesiologists, and surgeons, experienced with pediatric airway management. Age-appropriate size rigid bronchoscopes and optical foreign body forceps should be available.

## Esophageal Foreign Body

The incidence of foreign body ingestion is highest in children between the ages of 6 months and 6 years. The most common esophageal foreign body reported in the United States is a coin. The majority of children presenting after esophageal foreign body ingestion are not in acute distress. Patients may be completely asymptomatic or complain of dysphagia and decreased oral intake. Rarely, esophageal foreign bodies have been reported to cause airway obstruction through external compression of the trachea and inflammation [14]. These children may show signs of respiratory distress including drooling, tachypnea, and cyanosis.

In addition to a complete history and physical examination, children with suspected foreign body ingestion should undergo anterior/posterior (AP) and lateral chest X-rays. The majority of esophageal foreign bodies are radiopaque and will thus be visible on chest plain films. A two view chest X-ray is essential in helping to distinguish between a coin and a disc or "button" battery. In cases of an ingested disc battery, a "double ring" sign may be apparent on an AP chest film. On a lateral view, a disc battery appears as bilaminar with a "two-step border." This is in contrast to coins which have a smooth border on lateral films (Fig. **1**).

Esophageal foreign bodies are removed by rigid or flexible esophagoscopy. The majority of esophageal foreign bodies can be removed electively, usually within 12 hours of presentation. However, in children with suspected disc battery ingestion, the foreign body must be removed emergently. Disc batteries are now commonly found in many household electronics such as cameras and hearing aids. Disc batteries can result in alkaline chemical burns due to sodium hydroxide generated from the battery current. In the upper aerodigestive tract, ingestion of the 20-mm lithium disk battery has been associated with the most severe complications including esophageal perforation. Significant esophageal burns can occur as soon as 2 to 2.5 hours following ingestion [15].

## Ear and Nose Foreign Body

Ear and nose foreign bodies are a frequent occurrence in the pediatric population. Common foreign bodies that are clinically encountered include toys, food, paper, beads, and cotton. Ear foreign bodies are often asymptomatic and may be noted during a routine otologic examination. Children with ear foreign bodies may also present with aural fullness, pruritus, and ottorhea. Children with nasal foreign bodies frequently present with nasal obstruction and unilateral, foul-smelling nasal drainage. Epistaxis may also be reported.

The majority of ear and nose foreign bodies may be removed in the office setting electively. However, this should only be attempted by providers experienced in foreign body removal as repeated, failed attempts may cause swelling and trauma. Specialized otologic instruments such as a mastoid hook/seeker or a cupped forceps may facilitate ear foreign body removal. Topical nasal decongestants such as oxymetazoline are useful in removal of nasal foreign bodies. Children in whom the foreign body is suspected to be either a disc battery or a live insect should be referred for immediate removal. Children that cannot tolerate removal of the foreign body in the clinic setting may require an anesthetic.

## EPISTAXIS

In childhood, 90% of epistaxis originates from the anterior nasal septum. Most cases are self-limited or resolve with a short duration of external compression. Topical vasoconstrictors, such as 0.05% oxymetazoline, may also be utilized to treat an acute episode of epistaxis. Keeping the nasal mucosa moist through interventions such as Vaseline to the nasal sill and nasal saline spray can help to prevent epistaxis in prone children. Children with refractory epistaxis may necessitate referral to an otolaryngologist. Rarely, such patients may have an underlying coagulopathy or nasal mass that is contributing to the persistent epistaxis.

The initial step in the evaluation of the patient with acute epistaxis is identification of the source of bleeding. The provider should wear a headlight when examining the child so that both hands are free. Upright positioning reduces venous pressure and may assist in visualization. After a decongestant is applied, a nasal speculum and a small caliber suction should be utilized to gently remove all clots from the nasal passages. A prominent vessel is frequently identified on the anterior septum that can be cauterized with silver nitrate. Infrequently, nasal packing is required to achieve control of the epistaxis. Uncooperative patients or those with refractory epistaxis may require examination in the operating room.

## ACKNOWLEDGEMENT

Declared none.

## CONFLICT OF INTEREST

The authors have no conflicts of interest or financial disclosures.

## REFERENCES

[1]    Pediatric Advanced Life Support Course Guide & Pediatric Advanced Life Support Provider Manual. 2006. AHA

[2]    Hartnick JC, Cotton RT. Stridor and airway obstruction. In: Bluestone C, eds. Pediatric Otolaryngology. 4th ed. Philadelphia, PA: WB Saunders Co; 2003:1437-1447.

[3]    Guldfred LA, Lyhne D, Becker BC. Acute epiglottitis: epidemiology, clinical presentation, management and outcome. J Laryngol Otol. 2008;122(8):818-23.

[4]    Tibballs J, Watson T. Symptoms and signs differentiating croup and epiglottitis. J Paediatr Child Health. 2011;47(3):77-82. doi:10.1111/j.1440-1754.2010.01892.x

[5]    Salamone FN, Bobbitt DB, Myer CM, Rutter MJ, Greinwald JH Jr. Bacterial tracheitis reexamined: is there a less severe manifestation?. Otolaryngol Head Neck Surg. 2004;131(6):871-6.

[6]    Tebruegge M, Pantazidou A, Thorburn K, *et al.* Bacterial tracheitis: a multi-centre perspective. Scand J Infect Dis. 2009;41(8):548-57.

[7]    Huang YL, Peng CC, Chiu NC, *et al.* Bacterial tracheitis in pediatrics: 12 year experience at a medical center in Taiwan. Pediatr Int. 2009;51(1):110-3.

[8]    Pearson SE, Rimell FR, Sidman J. Injuries to the Lower Respiratory Tract In: Bluestone C, eds. Pediatric Otolaryngology. 4th ed. Philadelphia, PA: WB Saunders Co; 2003:1511-1518.

[9]    Pierrot S, Bernardeschi D, Morrisseau-Durand MP, Manach Y, Couloigner V. Dissection of the internal carotid artery following trauma of the soft palate in children. Ann Otol Rhinol Laryngol. 2006;115(5):323-9.

[10]   Soose RJ, Simons JP, Mandell DL. Evaluation and management of pediatric oropharyngeal trauma. Arch Otolaryngol Head Neck Surg. 2006;132(4):446-51.

[11]   Fagan P, Patel N. A hole in the drum. An overview of tympanic membrane perforations. Aust Fam Physician. 2002;31(8):707-10.

[12]   Rimell FL, Thome A Jr, Stool S, *et al.* Characteristics of objects that cause choking in children. JAMA. 1995;274(22):1763-6.

[13]   Even L, *et al.* Diagnostic evaluation of foreign body aspiration in children: a prospective study. Journal of Pediatric Surgery (2005) 40, 1122-27.

[14]   Kim N, Atkinson N, Manicone P. Esophageal foreign body: a case of a neonate with stridor. Pediatr Emerg Care. 2008;24(12):849-51.

[15]   Litovitz T, Whitaker N, Clark L, White NC, Marsolek M. Emerging battery-ingestion hazard: clinical implications. Pediatrics. 2010;125(6):1168-77.

Send Orders of Reprints at reprints@benthamscience.net

# CHAPTER 8

## Pediatric Cervical/Deep Neck Space Infections

## Stanley Voigt[1] and Jan C. Groblewski[1,2,*]

*[1]Department of Otolaryngology, Tufts University Medical Center, Boston, MA, USA and [2]Division of Otolaryngology, Warren Alpert Medical School of Brown University, Providence, RI, USA*

**Abstract:** Deep neck space infections (DNSI) are common in the pediatric population but frequently present diagnostic and management challenges for the practitioner. If undiagnosed or inappropriately managed, infections of the deep neck can progress rapidly and cause significant morbidity and mortality. In this chapter, relevant anatomy, etiology, pathophysiology, clinical presentation, diagnosis, medical and surgical management, and potential complications are discussed.

**Keywords:** Neck abscess, Neck infection, Deep neck space infection, Parapharyngeal abscess, Retropharyngeal abscess, Danger space, mediastinitis, peritonsillar abscess, ludwigs, lemierre's syndrome, MRSA, Carotid artery aneurysm.

### ANATOMY OF DEEP NECK SPACES

Knowledge of the fascial planes and spaces of the neck is paramount in the management of patients with DNSI. The cervical fascia separates the neck into potential spaces. This fascia is divided into the Superficial and Deep Cervical fascia. The Superficial Cervical fascia lies just deep to the dermis and encases the platysma muscle. The Deep Cervical fascia is further subdivided into three layers. The Superficial (anterior) investing layer of the Deep Cervical fascia completely encircles the neck and passes anterior to the trapezius and sternocleidomastoid muscles. The middle layer of the deep cervical fascia has two subdivisions: the muscular and visceral fascia. The muscular division surrounds the strap muscles and is continuous with the superficial layer at the lateral borders of these muscles. The visceral division surrounds the trachea, thyroid gland and esophagus. This division contributes superiorly to the buccopharyngeal fascia. The deep layer of the Deep Cervical fascia, which is also known as the prevertebral fascia, consists of two divisons anteromedially, the alar and prevertebral divisons [1, 2].

*Address correspondence to Jan Groblewski: Division of Otolaryngology, Warren Alpert Medical School of Brown University, Boston, MA, USA; Tel: 401.274.2300; Fax: 401.272.1302; E-mail: jgroblewski@lifespan.org

These Deep Cervical fascial planes separate the neck into potential spaces. These spaces can communicate with one another but are divided anatomically. The retropharyngeal space lies between the visceral layer of the middle layer and the alar division of the deep layer. The inferior extent of this space is the mediastinum and superiorly it extends to the skull base [1]. This space contains the retropharyngeal lymph nodes.

The parapharyngeal space is described as an "inverted pyramid" that is located lateral to the upper pharynx [1]. Its boundaries include the pterygomandibular raphe anteriorly, the prevertebral space posteriorly, the superior constrictor muscle medially, and the mandible and lateral pterygoid muscle laterally. This space is in close relation to the retropharyngeal space and infections can easily penetrate through the loose fascia that separates these two spaces [2].

The so-called 'Danger' space is a potential space of loose connective tissue between the alar and prevertebral divisions of the deep layer of the Deep Cervical fascia. It extends from the skull base superiorly to the diaphragm inferiorly, and allows for rapid transmission of infection to the posterior mediastinum. In relation to the other neck spaces it is located between the retropharyngeal and prevertebral spaces [1].

The peritonsillar space is a potential space between the superior constrictor muscle and the capsule of the palatine tonsil. The submandibular space spans from the floor of mouth superiorly to the superficial layer of the Deep Cervical fascia as it extends from the hyoid bone to mandible superiorly. This space is subdivided by the mylohyoid muscle into a superior sublingual compartment and an inferior submaxillary compartment [1, 2]. The prevertebral space sits anterior to the vertebral bodies and posterior to the prevertebral division of the deep layer of the Deep Cervical fascia. It extends from the base of skull to the coccyx.

## ETIOLOGY & MICROBIOLOGY

DNSI in children are most commonly caused by upper respiratory infections such as tonsillitis or pharyngitis. Odontogenic infections, salivary gland infections, and rhinosinusitis are less common etiologies. Additional potential causes to consider include dental procedures, trauma, foreign body aspiration, and congenital neck cysts. Typically, bacterial pathogens associated with the primary infection will travel *via* the lymphatic system to the deep lymph nodes of the neck, most commonly the parapharyngeal and retropharyngeal nodes. The retropharyngeal space tends to be involved in younger children since most retropharyngeal lymph nodes involute after 5 years of age [3]. Once deep neck space lymph nodes are infected, the process can progress from cellulitis to phlegmon to mature abscess formation.

Deep neck space infections are typically polymicrobial, involving both anaerobic and aerobic species from the oral cavity and oropharyngeal flora. Anaerobic bacteria are 10 times more common as a source of infection than aerobic bacteria; however, the majority of oropharyngeal abscesses yield cultures that are polymicrobial [4]. The predominant anaerobic bacteria in the oropharyngeal flora causing DNSI are Fusobacterium, Prevotella, Porphyromonas & Peptostreptococcus spp. The most common aerobic bacteria are *Staphylococcus aureus*, *Streptococcus pyogenes* & *Haemophilus influenzae*. Retropharyngeal abscesses are more likely to harbor aerobic organisms (Groups A & B Streptoccocus and *Staphylococcus aureus*). *Fusobacterium necrophorum* can be associated with the development of septic thrombophlebitis in Lemierre's. Rare sources of DNSI include *Mycobacterium tuberculosis*, Atypical *Mycobacterium*, *Coccidioides immitis* and even *Bartonella henselae* [4, 5].

In recent years there has been a general rise in the frequency of DNSI caused by methicillin-resistant Staphylococcus aureus (MRSA), particularly in the pediatric population. These patients typically have community acquired MRSA (CA-MRSA). This trend has implications for the treatment of DNSI because antimicrobial therapy is routinely started prior to the retrieval of cultures. Coverage to include CA-MRSA must be considered in light of this trend, especially when patients are not responsive to initial antibiotics [6].

## CLINICAL PRESENTATION

The clinical presentation of children with DNSI is dependent on many factors, including preceding treatment with oral antibiotics, patient age, the location of the infection, and the presence or absence of associated systemic symptoms or complications. Most children who present with a DNSI have had preceding upper respiratory symptoms for approximately 5 days in duration and have already been treated with oral antibiotics [7].

The most common symptoms at the time of presentation are fever and neck pain. Children may also have neck stiffness, swelling, dysphagia, odynophagia, trismus, or, in rare occasions, upper respiratory obstruction with difficulty breathing. In this section we will briefly describe the common types of DNSI affecting children and their typical presentations [7].

**Parapharyngeal:** Children with parapharyngeal DNSI commonly present with fever, odynophagia & dysphagia. On exam patients may be found to have a bulge in the lateral pharyngeal wall along with medial displacement of the tonsil. They also may be found to have a unilateral neck mass or neck fullness [7].

**Retropharyngeal:** DNSI involving the retropharyngeal space tend to affect children who are younger than 5 years of age. Common presenting signs and symptoms are sometimes nonspecific but may include fever, irritability, drooling and decreased oral intake. Signs of more advanced disease may include stridor, obstructive sleep apnea, or even respiratory distress.

**Peritonsillar:** Peritonsillar infections are most common in the adolescent or young adult population, who may complain of fever, odynophagia, dysphagia, and trismus, and who may have also experienced a voice change (classically the 'hot potato voice'). On exam, patients often have contralateral uvular deviation, unilateral medialization of the tonsil and erythema and edema of the affected anterior tonsillar pillar [7].

**Ludwigs:** Recently it has been reported that 27 to 50% of those affected by Ludwigs are children [8, 9]. These patients typically present with neck pain, fever, odynophagia, dysphagia, and drooling. They may also have tooth pain, trismus, or voice changes. On physical examination children with Ludwigs can be found to have extensive neck swelling in the submental and submandibular regions, and may also have induration of the floor of mouth. If the disease process has progressed further by the time of presentation, patients can also have symptoms of airway obstruction including dyspnea or stridor [8].

## DIAGNOSIS

Physical examination: In general, most children with DNSI will have neck swelling and an elevated temperature. Neck swelling is sometimes generalized, without confined areas of fluctuance as is often noted in more superficial infections. Neck mobility is typically decreased and should also be assessed. Additional physical examination findings that can be seen in patients with a DNSI include trismus, oropharyngeal asymmetry, retropharyngeal bulging, and dental tenderness.

**Labwork:** A complete blood count (CBC) with emphasis on the white blood cell count is essential upon presentation, as these patients typically display a leukocytosis. However, values must be obtained with a full understanding of the patient's medical history because those patients with viral illness, immunodeficiency or tumor may not mount this response. In addition, patients who have received steroids may display a steroid-related leukocytosis making true determination of their white blood cell count difficult. This should not prohibit obtaining a daily CBC as these values can be trended regardless [1]. Blood cultures should also be obtained at the time of presentation to rule out bacteremia.

**Imaging:** Plain radiographs are rapid and inexpensive and can provide diagnostic information in selected DNSI. If a retropharyngeal abscess is suspected, a lateral neck radiograph is a valuable screening image that may demonstrate thickening of the retropharyngeal soft tissue (Fig. **1**). If there is greater than 5mm of thickening at the level of C2 or an air-fluid level in the retropharyngeal space, there is a very strong likelihood of a retropharyngeal infection. The major limitation of plain radiographs is their inability to discern between cellulitis and abscess. As a result, a lower threshold for obtaining CT scans is now advocated [10].

Ultrasound is a non-invasive and inexpensive modality that is becoming a more popular imaging choice in the evaluation of DNSI. In the pediatric population, where there are concerns for radiation and sedation for CT and MRI, respectively, ultrasound can be an excellent alternative. Ultrasonography can also aid practitioners with image guidance for needle aspiration of abscesses for culture and therapeutic relief in certain cases. The limitations of ultrasound include the inability to adequately image the retrophyarnx and the inability to appropriately assess the extent of significant infections where the cavity may extend beyond its focal range [1].

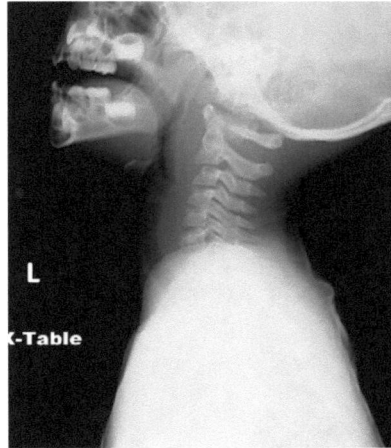

**Figure 1:** Standard lateral neck X-ray demonstrating significant retropharyngeal thickening in a 3.5-year-old girl.

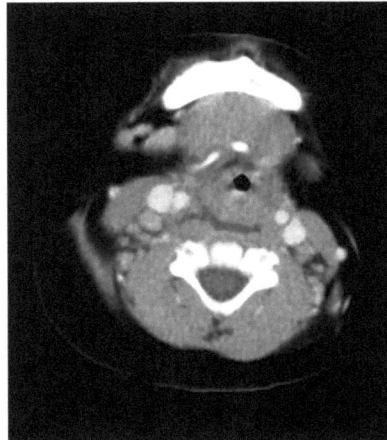

**Figure 2:** Axial CT scan with contrast demonstrating a retropharyngeal fluid collection extending to the lower level of the hypopharynx in a 6.5-month-old boy.

Computed tomography (CT) is the imaging modality of choice in the evaluation of DNSI. The usefulness of CT imaging is in its ability not only to specifically localize the source of infection but also to aid in the determination of whether the infectious process has progressed along the spectrum from cellulitis to phlegmon to abscess (Fig. **2**). Many advocate for an initial CT upon presentation. If a conservative treatment approach is followed, CT may be indicated 24 to 48 hours after the initiation of intravenous antibiotics to determine if a previously noted cellulitis or phlegmon has formed into an abscess, which often dictates the need for surgical intervention (Fig. **3**) [8]. CT is particularly important in surgical decision-making and often helps the otolaryngologist determine whether an abscess will be best accessed trans-orally or trans-cervically.

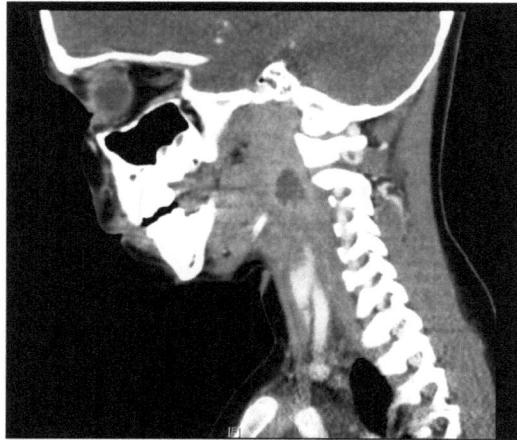

**Figure 3:** Sagittal CT scan with contrast demonstrating a left parapharyngeal abscess in a 5-year-old girl. Note the proximity of the abscess to the prevertebral and 'Danger' spaces.

CT scan should always be performed with contrast when evaluating children with possible DNSI. Certain characteristics, including low attenuation fluid with low Houndsfield units and contrast enhancement of the surrounding tissue, are strongly suggestive that the patient has an abscess (Fig. **4**). The accuracy of CT in distinguishing true abscess from phlegmon varies from source to source, with some sources citing accuracy as low as 63%. However, other sources demonstrated a 95% sensitivity of CT scanning with contrast for DNSI [8].

The risk of radiation exposure on children has been a source of great debate, but should always be considered when managing patients with DNSI. Studies show that the use of CT has increased seven times compared to the 1980's [11]. Children are more sensitive to radiation than adults and given their longer life expectancy they have a larger window of time to express radiation damage [11].

CT imaging should therefore not be used excessively to monitor patients unless clinical examination is uncertain.

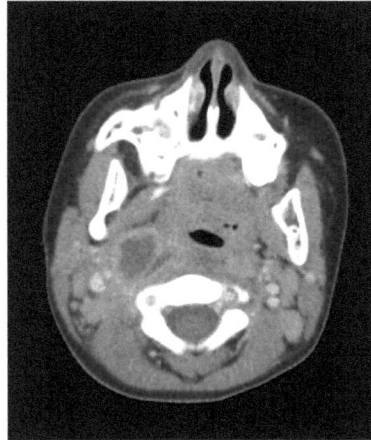

**Figure 4:** Axial CT scan with contrast demonstrating a right parapharyngeal abscess in a 6-year-old girl. Note the contrast enhancement of the tissue surrounding the abscess.

Magnetic Resonance Imaging (MRI) has a very limited role in the evaluation of DNSI. This modality is typically reserved for those who have contraindications to CT because it is time consuming, not as cost-effective, and requires more patience on the part of the child or adolescent if sedation is not being used. MR angiography can be very useful in the evaluation of pseudoaneurysms or thrombi [1].

## MANAGEMENT

Initial management of patients with DNI involves clinical evaluation of the patient's airway. The airway should first be secured and then maintained. Most patients need humidified air only, whereas others with mild or moderate airway symptoms may benefit from intravenous steroids or treatment with racemic epinephrine. If there is any significant concern regarding the patient's airway, an urgent Pediatric Otolaryngology and anesthesia evaluation may be necessary. The otolaryngology evaluation may include flexible laryngoscopy, which allows visualization of the upper airway and can help dictate patient management [1]. Rarely do pediatric patients with deep neck abscesses undergo tracheostomy, however the threshold for otolaryngology involvement in the initial evaluation should be low [7]. Once the airway is properly addressed, intravenous hydration and intravenous antibiotics should be initiated. Maintenance fluids are imperative as children often have limited oral intake due to pain with swallowing and are therefore at a higher risk for dehydration [1]. Initial intravenous antibiotics will typically have gram positive and anaerobic coverage, such as Clindamycin or Ampicillin-Sulbactam [12]. Clindamycin offers great sensitivity even to pediatric patients with suspected CA-MRSA [6].

Surgical drainage maintains an important role in the management of patients with DNSI. In general, surgical drainage is indicated in children with large abscesses or associated complications, or when there is a lack of clinical response to conservative therapy over a 48-72 hour period and a purulent fluid collection has been identified. Surgical consultation with Pediatric Otolaryngology is recommended early in the natural history of a DNSI to determine the need for incision and drainage. Children who present with phelgmon or cellulitis should be managed initially with intravenous antibiotics alone. In addition, patients with small abscesses less than 2cm$^3$ may respond to intravenous antibiotics only [8, 13].

Surgical management, when necessary, typically consists of formal incision and drainage under general anesthesia. There are many surgical approaches to deep neck space abscesses and decisions regarding what approach is appropriate depend on many factors, primarily the location and extent of the abscess. Incision and drainage is typically performed transcervically or transorally, and involves wide opening of the abscess cavity followed by thorough debridement and irrigation. Some adolescent patients with peritonsillar abscess may tolerate bedside transoral incision and drainage procedures. Needle drainage of deep neck abscesses, with or without image guidance, has a limited role in these patients, but can be considered for obtaining cultures or when abscess location precludes safe incision and drainage [8].

## COMPLICATIONS FROM DEEP NECK SPACE INFECTIONS

The timely diagnosis and management of DNSI is imperative in order to prevent the morbidity and mortality associated with potential complications. Several factors have been shown to increase the risk of complications from DNSI, including younger age at presentation, retropharyngeal location and abscess cultures positive for *Staphylococcus Aureus* [14]. Also, there are regional variations in antibiotic susceptibility patterns, which can increase the risk of developing a complication if the initial infection is improperly treated. This highlights the importance of the provider being aware of the susceptibility profiles of their hospital prior to initiating treatment. Potential complications from DNSI include bacteremia/sepsis, airway compromise, mediastinitis, Lemierre's syndrome and carotid artery aneurysm or rupture [14].

**Airway Compromise:** Due to the location of the deep neck spaces, children with DNSI can be at risk for airway compromise. If there is concern for impending airway compromise, or if the patient presents with airway symptoms, the patient should be monitored in an intensive care setting. Initial airway therapy may include oxygenated face tent with cool mist humidity, intravenous steroids, or inhaled racemic epinephrine. Some children will need to be intubated, and in very rare cases some may require urgent tracheostomy. Patients with concern for airway compromise require involvement of both Pediatric Otolaryngology and anesthesiology/critical care services [1].

**Mediastinitis:** One of the most concerning complications of DNSI is mediastinitis, which has a high mortality rate of 30-40% [15]. All DNSI can propagate *via* deep neck spaces and spread to the upper mediastinum, leading to mediastinitis. These patients may have symptoms of tachycardia, hypoxia, dyspnea, and pleuritic pain. They sometimes exhibit diffuse neck edema on examination. Any concern for developing mediastinitis should prompt a chest radiograph, which may show characteristic mediastinal widening or pleural effusions. Multiple organisms are typically involved in mediastinitis so broad spectrum IV antibiotic coverage is necessary to include gram-positive, gram-negative, aerobic, and anaerobic species. Surgical management is essential and is dependent on the degree of involvement of the mediastinum. If the process is limited to the anterior-superior mediastinum, transcervical drainage may be sufficient. If the infection includes more than one mediastinal compartment, a thoracotomy is typically performed in addition to the transcervical drainage [1].

**Lemierre's Disease:** Lemierre's is characterized by internal jugular vein thrombophlebitis and gram-negative sepsis. The pathogen involved in the development of this disease is *Fusobacterium Necrophorum*, an anaerobic bacteria that is part of the normal orophargyngeal flora. This uncommon complication is thought to arise from invasion of the bacterium from the oropharynx through tonsillar veins into the internal jugular venous system, where platelet aggregation is induced *via* bacterial endotoxin [1]. This induces septic thrombus formation, which can embolize to the lungs and the joints. The typical presentation is that of a young male who presents following a recent pharyngitis with acute onset of fever, rigors, tachycardia, hypoxia and lateral neck tenderness and edema. These patients may also exhibit dyspnea & pleuritic chest pain as 97% of these patients will develop septic pulmonary emboli during their hospital course [16]. CT of the neck will reveal a filling defect of the internal jugular venous system. Treatment involves a prolonged course of beta-lactamase resistant IV antibiotics as there appears to be increasing beta-lactamase positivity in the *Fusobacterium* organism. The role of anticoagulation and duration of therapy remains controversial and recommendations range from no anticoagulation to up to 6 months of anticoagulation with Coumadin. The goal of anticoagulation is to prevent retrograde thrombophlebitis extending to the intracranial sinuses. Some advocate short-term anticoagulation with discontinuation several days after resolution of the acute illness [16].

Carotid Artery Aneurysm or Rupture: The treatment of Deep Neck Space infections with antibiotics has drastically reduced the incidence of vascular complications since the early 1900's. Carotid artery aneurysm is a rare complication of DNSI and often poses a significant challenge to an unsuspecting provider who has had minimal experience with its diagnosis or treatment. This complication can result from the spread of the DNSI from the retropharyngeal or parapharyngeal spaces into the carotid space. Clinical findings that should lead one to suspect that the infection may involve the extra-cranial carotid arteries include bright red recurrent oropharyngeal bleeding, an expanding pulsatile neck mass, or a cervical bruit or thrill. This life-threatening complication requires ligation of the common carotid artery without delay and literature in children has shown that this procedure often results in little if any neurologic sequelae [17].

## ACKNOWLEDGEMENT

Declared none.

## CONFLICT OF INTEREST

The author(s) confirm that this chapter content has no conflict of interest.

## REFERENCES

[1]     Oliver ER & Gillespie MB. Deep Neck Space Infections. In: Flint PW, Bruce HH *et al.* *Cummings Otolaryngology: Head & Neck Surgery*, fifth edition. Philadelphia: Mosby Inc., 2010.

[2]     Hollinshead WH. Fascia and Fascial Spaces of the Head and Neck. *Anatomy for Surgeons*, Volume 2. London: Cassell & Co, 1956.

[3]     Pappas DE & Hendley JO. Retropharyngeal Abscess, Lateral Pharyngeal Abscesss, and Peritonsillar Cellulitis/Abscess. In: Kleighman RM *et al.* *Nelson Textbook of Pediatrics*, 19th ed. Philadelphia PA: W.B. Saunders, 2011.

[4]     Brook I. Microbiology and Management of Peritonsillar, Retropharyngeal, and Parapharyngeal Abscesses. *Journal of Oral and Maxillofacial Surgery*. 2004; 62: 1545- 1550.

[5]     Yeh SH, Zangwill KM *et al.* Parapharyngeal Abscess Due to Cat-Scratch Disease. *Clinical Infectious Diseases*. 2000; 30(3): 599-601.

[6]     Ossowski K, Chun R *et al.* Increased Isolation of Methicillin-Resistant Staphylococcus Aureus in Pediatric Head and Neck Abscesses. *Archives of Otolaryngology Head and Neck Surgery*. 2006; 132: 1176-1181.

[7]     Herzon FS & Martin AD. Medical and Surgical Treatment of Peritonsillar, Retropharyngeal, and parapharyngeal Abscesses. *Current Infectious Disease Reports.* 2006; 8(3): 196-202.

[8]     Nagy M, Pizzuto M *et al.* Deep Neck Infections in Children: A New Approach to Diagnosis and Treatment. *The Laryngoscope.* 1997; 107: 1627-1634.

[9]     Lin HW, O'Neill A *et al.* Ludwig's Angina in the Pediatric Population. Clinical Pediatrics. 2009; 48:583-587.

[10]    Uzomefuna V, Glynn F *et al.* Atypical Locations of Retropharygeal Abscess: Beware of the Normal Lateral Soft Tissue Neck X-Ray. *International Journal of Pediatric Otorhinolaryngology.* 2010; 74: 1445-1448.

[11]    Bajohli M, Bajoghli F *et al.* Children, CT Scan and Radiation. *International Journal of Preventive Medicine.* 2010; 1(4): 220-222.

[12]    Chang L, Chi H *et al.* Deep Neck Infections in Different Age Groups of Children. *Journal of Microbiology, Immunology and Infection.* 2010; 43(1):47-52.134.

[13]    McClay JE, Murray AD, Booth T. Intravenous Antibiotic Therapy for deep neck abscesses defined by computed tomography. *Arch Otolaryngol Head Neck Surg.* 2003; 129: 1207- 1212.

[14]    Baldassari CM, Howell R *et al.* Complications in pediatric deep neck space abscesses. Otolaryngol Head Neck Surg. 2011; 144(4): 592-595.

[15]    Shah RK, Chun R, Choi SS. Mediastinitis in infants from deep neck space infections. *Otolaryngol Head Neck Surg,* 2009;140(6):936-8.

[16]    Bondy P & Grant T. Lemierre's Syndrome: What Are the Roles for Anticoagulation and Long-Term Antibiotic Therapy? *Annals of Otology, Rhinology & Laryngology.* 2008; 117(9): 679-683.

[17]    Lueg EA, Awerbuck D *et al.* Ligation of the Common Carotid Artery for the Management of a Mycotic Pseudoaneurysm of an extracranial internal carotid artery. A case report and review of the literature. *Int Journal of Pediatric Otorhinolarynglogy.* 1995; 33: 67-74.

# CHAPTER 9

## Pediatric Stridor

## Joshua R. Bedwell and George H. Zalzal[*]

*Children's National Medical Center, George Washington University, 111 Michigan Avenue, NW, Washington, D.C. 20010, USA*

**Abstract:** Stridor is noisy breathing due to airway obstruction, and may be caused by a vast array of pathologies. Children present with stridor along a continuum of acuity and severity. Causes of acute stridor include infections and foreign bodies. Chronic stridor may be due to a wide array of functional and anatomic anomalies, with common causes including laryngomalacia, recurrent respiratory papillomatosis, subglottic stenosis, vocal fold paralysis, and airway hemangioma. Laryngomalacia is far and away the most common cause for chronic stridor in the infant.

In order to correctly diagnose and manage the stridulous child, a detailed history regarding the onset, progression, and nature of the stridor, and a thorough physical examination, potentially including laryngoscopy must be performed. Management must start with ensuring a safe and secure airway, followed by correction of the underlying cause.

**Keywords:** Stridor, airway, laryngotracheitis, croup, epiglottitis, bacterial tracheitis, airway foreign body, laryngomalacia, recurrent respiratory papillomatosis, subglottic stenosis, vocal fold paralysis, vocal cord paralysis, hemangioma, laryngoscopy, bronchoscopy, supraglottoplasty, tracheotomy.

## INTRODUCTION

Stridor is a frequently encountered physical exam finding that may be caused by a vast array of pathologies. Simply put, stridor is noisy breathing that arises from turbulent airflow caused by airway obstruction. In the already small pediatric airway, tiny impingements on the lumen can create large increases in resistance.

[*]**Address correspondence to George H. Zalzal:** Children's National Medical Center, 111 Michigan Avenue, NW, Washington, D.C. 20010, USA; Tel: 202 476-3852; Fax: 202 476-5038; E-mail: gzalzal@cnmc.org

This is explained by Poiseuille's law, which states that flow is inversely proportional to the fourth power of the radius.

Stridor should be differentiated from stertor. Typically, stridor is described as a high-pitched noise, though it can vary widely in pitch and quality. Stertor is a low-pitched, snoring sound typically caused by obstruction at the nasal, nasopharyngeal, or oropharyngeal level. Stridor, on the other hand, is more commonly found with supraglottic, glottic, or subglottic obstruction.

## PRESENTATION AND PHYSICAL EXAM

Children present with stridor along a continuum of acuity and severity. At one end of the spectrum lies the stridulous child in acute respiratory distress, and at the other, the otherwise asymptomatic child who is noted to "squeak" a bit when feeding. In any child presenting in acute distress, the establishment of a safe and secure airway is paramount. Important historical points that may be quickly elucidated to aid in determining the safest management of the airway include the presence of trauma, suspicion of foreign body ingestion or aspiration, or signs and symptoms of acute infection (fever, malaise, *etc.*). In most cases, it is prudent to defer any invasive physical examination of such children until in the operating room with airway instruments at the ready. In a stable child, a more complete history may be obtained, and in general there are several crucial points that can aid in narrowing the diagnosis. Table **1** lists relevant history and physical points.

**Table 1:** Important History and Physical Examination Points.

| History | Physical Exam |
|---|---|
| Onset | Respiratory rate/Work of breathing |
| Progression | Weight (Failure to thrive) |
| Exacerbating factors (*i.e.* position, feeding) | Characteristics of stridor: inspiratory/expiratory/biphasic |
| Cyanotic events/ALTEs | Suprasternal/Substernal/Intercostal retractions |
| Feeding problems | Flaring of alae nasi<br>Tripod positioning/neck extension |
| Hoarse voice/weak cry | Syndromic facies/craniofacial anomalies (*i.e.* retrognathia, macroglossia, *etc.*) |
| Witnessed choking episode (foreign body) | Auscultation of neck/chest |
| Signs of infection (fever, malaise, *etc.*) | Neck masses/fullness |
| Prior intubation | Complete ENT examination |
| Prior cardiac surgery | |

Comorbidities (*i.e.* Arnold-Chiari malformation, craniofacial anomalies, cutaneous hemangiomas, *etc.*)

The age of onset is an important clue. Stridor apparent from the time of birth commonly points toward a congenital anatomic abnormality, such as a glottic web, subglottic or tracheal stenosis, or a vocal cord paralysis. The characteristic inspiratory stridor of laryngomalacia may be present at birth, or may appear in the early post-natal period. Stridor that worsens over time may indicate a growing lesion, such as a vallecular cyst, hemangioma, subglottic cyst, or external compression from a mediastinal mass or vascular sling. Worsening stridor over time may also be due to increased physical exertion by a growing child.

Exacerbating factors should be probed. Symptoms may be positional in nature: children with laryngomalacia or obstruction from a malpositioned tongue base (*i.e.* from craniofacial anomalies such as Pierre-Robin sequence) often have more severe symptoms when supine, and will improve with side or prone positioning. Vascular lesions may engorge with crying or straining, leading to worsened stridor.

Close attention to associated signs and symptoms can help define the severity of the underlying condition, as well as narrow the differential diagnosis. Episodes of cyanosis, or "apparent life threatening events" (ALTEs) are a troubling sign that should prompt immediate workup, including a cardiologic evaluation. Gastroesophageal reflux can exacerbate underlying airway anomalies, as well as cause laryngeal irritation that can present as stridor, and the clinician should inquire about a history of frequent reflux or regurgitation. Children with airway obstruction may also present with feeding difficulties. Commonly reported issues include: slow feeding, coughing, choking, regurgitation, and feeding intolerance. Such problems can lead to poor weight gain, and in severe cases, failure to thrive.

Other potential sequelae involve consequences of prolonged severe airway obstruction. Pectus excavatum has been a known complication since as early as 1897, when Sutherland and Lack described the natural history of children with congenital stridor. Cor pulmonale is a potentially fatal development, and a definite indication for surgical management. Two pathways are implicated in its evolution: chronic hypoxia leading to polycythemia and increased blood viscosity, and hypercapnea leading to pulmonary hypertension [1].

While it is an important part of the history in general, a detailed perinatal history, with attention to a history of prior intubation is key in the evaluation of the stridulous child. Depending on the time that has passed from extubation to the presentation of stridor, one may suspect granuloma, vocal cord immobility, or, further on from extubation, subglottic stenosis.

A detailed accounting of the past medical history is important as there are numerous medical conditions, craniofacial anomalies, and syndromes that can be associated with airway abnormalities. While a complete list is beyond the scope of this chapter, some of the more common ones are listed in Table **2**.

**Table 2:** Notable Medical Comorbidities Associated with Airway Anomalies

| |
|---|
| Arnold-Chiari Malformation |
| Craniofacial Syndromes:<br>• Treacher-Collins<br>• Pierre-Robin<br>• Apert<br>• Crouzon |
| Down syndrome |
| CHARGE Syndrome |
| PHACES Syndrome |
| 22q11 deletion/DiGeorge/Velo-Cardio-Facial Syndrome |

Physical examination of the stable child with stridor should begin with an overall assessment of the child's appearance. The child's height and weight should be noted, and compared to a growth chart to evaluate for poor weight gain or failure to thrive. Tell-tale craniofacial abnormalities may indicate an underlying syndrome. The degree to which the child is working to breathe can be determined using parameters including the respiratory rate, use of accessory muscles, and suprasternal and/or intercostal retractions. The child's vocal quality can be an important clue as to etiology. A hoarse or aphonic cry may indicate a vocal fold paralysis, or other anatomic abnormality at the glottic level, although children with an immobile vocal fold often have normal voices. A complete head and neck exam is essential, noting findings that may contribute to airway obstruction, including micro/retrognathia, macroglossia, tonsillar hypertrophy, and the presence of any palpable neck masses.

Both the chest and neck should be auscultated. The phase or phases of respiration in which the stridor is present often points to the level of obstruction. Stridor noted during the inspiratory phase is typically seen with supraglottic pathologies. Expiratory stridor is frequently seen in tracheal lesions, such as tracheomalacia. Stridor present during both inspiration and expiration, described as biphasic stridor, connotes a fixed obstruction at the glottic or subglottic level.

## Further Workup

Radiologic studies can play a useful role in the evaluation of stridulous patients. AP and lateral X-rays of the chest and neck may identify subglottic or tracheal narrowing, or the presence of an aspirated or swallowed foreign body. CT scans of the neck and chest are used in the workup of patients with vascular slings to identify the nature of the vascular anomaly. Advanced reformatting of these CT images, such as 3-D reconstructions of the airway may be helpful in documenting the length of a narrowed tracheal segment. The barium esophagram may also demonstrate compression by a vascular ring, or can diagnose a tracheo-esophageal fistula. In patients for whom aspiration is a concern, a modified barium swallow may be indicated. Alternatively, a flexible endoscopic evaluation of swallowing (FEES) performed in conjunction with a speech and swallow therapist can be used in the appropriate patient. Often, patients with suspected GERD are treated empirically with either histamine receptor blockers or proton pump inhibitors. In those who do not respond, a 24-hour pH probe study may be of use.

## ENDOSCOPIC EVALUATION

An indispensable tool in the otolaryngologist's arsenal for evaluating the upper airway is the flexible fiberoptic laryngoscope. Flexible fiberoptic laryngoscopy (FFL) allows for complete evaluation of the airway from the nasal cavity, through the choanae into the nasopharynx and oropharynx, allowing an excellent view of the supraglottic and glottic larynx. This may be performed in the office, after applying a small amount of topical anesthesia to the nasal mucosa. It provides valuable information about both anatomic and functional abnormalities, as one can examine the child in an un-sedated state. One may note supralaryngeal anomalies such as prolapse of the tongue base posteriorly, vallecular cyst, or poor pharyngeal tone. An excellent view of the supraglottis and glottis is obtained. Occasionally, a view of the subglottis can be obtained, and obvious lesions (*i.e.* subglottic hemangioma) may be seen, though this area is best examined in the operating room with direct laryngoscopy and bronchoscopy.

With the child anesthetized in the operating room, direct laryngoscopy and bronchoscopy gives the surgeon a detailed view of the entire airway. Ideally done with the child spontaneously breathing, a laryngoscope is used to visualize the larynx, and topical lidocaine (4%) is sprayed over the laryngeal structures with a maximum dose of 5mg/kg. During the examination, oxygen is insufflated into the pharynx either *via* a side port on the laryngoscope, or nasotracheal tube situated in the pharynx. The airway may then be examined in detail from supraglottis to the mainstem bronchi, either with a ventilating bronchoscope outfitted with a 0-degree Hopkins rod, or with only the endoscope itself. Recent advances in high-definition cameras and monitors allow excellent visualization.

The subglottis can be sized with uncuffed endotracheal tubes to evaluate for the presence and severity of subglottic stenosis when suspected. The patient is orotracheally intubated and the positive pressure is given by the anesthesiologist to determine the presence of a leak (evaluated by visualizing the subglottis and examining for bubbling, and listening for an audible leak). The largest tube that allows an appropriate leak between 10-30cm water is noted (provided the subglottis is circular in shape). Subglottic narrowing due to an elliptically-shaped cricoid cartilage, or any other non-concentric narrowing should be identified and noted.

Direct laryngoscopy allows for the operative management of laryngeal and tracheal lesions. Using suspension laryngoscopes such as the Parsons or Lindholm allows the surgeon to have both hands free for instrumentation. A variety of tools are available for use in the airway, including cold-steel microlaryngoscopic instruments, the microdebrider, electrocautery, and the carbon dioxide laser.

## DIFFERENTIAL DIAGNOSIS

Appropriate management of the stridulous patient requires accurate diagnosis of the etiology of the stridor. Given the multitude of potential causes, one must approach the differential diagnosis in an organized fashion. Useful distinctions to make include acute onset *versus* chronic, congenital stridor *versus* acquired, and anatomic classifications of the pathology into supraglottic, glottic, subglottic, and tracheo-bronchial processes (Table **3**).

**Table 3:** Differential Diagnosis of Stridor.

|  | **Supraglottic** | **Glottic** | **Subglottic/Tracheal** |
|---|---|---|---|
| **Acute** | Foreign body | Foreign body | Foreign body |
|  | Epiglottitis | Trauma | Laryngotracheitis (Croup) Bacterial tracheitis |
| **Chronic** | Craniofacial anomalies | Vocal fold paralysis | Subglottic stenosis |
|  | Laryngomalacia | Intubation granuloma | Subglottic cyst |
|  | Recurrent Respiratory Papillomatosis | Laryngeal web | Hemangioma |
|  | Vallecular cyst | Partial laryngeal atresia | Vascular ring/sling |
|  | Hypotonia/Neurologic dysfunction |  | Complete tracheal rings |
|  |  |  | Extrinsic compression |

## Acute Onset

The most commonly encountered causes for acute onset stridor are infection and foreign body aspiration. Laryngotracheitis (croup) is the most common infectious cause of stridor in infants, and is typically seen in the 6 month to 2 year age frame. Parainfluenza virus is the most common infectious agent, though other viruses such as respiratory syncytial virus and rhinovirus are potential pathogens. These children present with stridor, typically biphasic in nature, accompanied by systemic signs of infection (fever, malaise). While the stridor can be impressive at times, these children rarely require intubation, and can be managed with humidification, systemic steroids, and racemic epinephrine nebulizer treatments as needed. Children with recurrent bouts of croup should be evaluated with direct laryngoscopy when healthy to rule out a pre-existing airway lesion.

In the modern era of *Haemophilus influenza* type B vaccinations, epiglottitis has become an exceedingly rare cause of acute onset stridor and airway compromise. Nevertheless, given the potentially disastrous consequences of mismanagement, it remains important to know the signs and symptoms and maintain a high index of suspicion for epiglottitis in the appropriate patient. These patients have an acute onset, and often rapid progression of fever, sore throat, drooling, muffled voice and inspiratory stridor. Physical examination and any invasive maneuver (placement of an intravenous line, blood draw) should be deferred until is in the operating room with all equipment necessary to secure the airway (including a tracheotomy tray) available.

Bacterial tracheitis is an exudative infection of the airway. Children present similar to those with croup, with stridor, systemic signs of infection, and often similar radiographic findings of subglottic narrowing. They often have a history of an antecedent viral upper respiratory tract infection. Bacterial tracheitis should be suspected in the child who does not respond to standard croup treatments, or worsens despite them. In such cases, airway endoscopy is indicated for diagnosis and culture of the exudates. Airway obstruction may occur due to edema, or secondary to displacement of tracheal pseudomembranes. In addition to diagnostic value, endoscopy allows suctioning and debridement of exudate. The pathogens responsible generally those typically seen in upper aerodigestive tract infections, including *Staphylococcus aureus*, *Streptococcus pneumonia*, Group A *Streptococcus*, and *Moraxella catarrhalis*. Treatment of these patients centers on adequate airway management, and systemic antibiotics.

Foreign body aspiration often presents with a history of a choking or coughing attack. A neck and chest X-ray can be helpful if the aspirated object is radioopaque. Evidence of bronchial obstruction by a radiolucent object can be obtained with inspiratory and expiratory films in a cooperative child, or lateral decubitus films in younger patients. The lung on the side of the foreign body may show signs of hyperinflation. However, normal X-rays in the face of a suspicious clinical picture should not prevent endoscopic evaluation in the operating room. An impacted esophageal object should also be ruled out, since edema may also impinge on the airway and lead to stridor.

## Chronic Stridor

Within the broad group of etiologies for subacute or chronic stridor, the differential can be narrowed by clarifying the age of onset of symptoms. Overall, congenital lesions are responsible for most cases of chronic stridor in children, around 84% of the time in one large series [2].

## *Laryngomalacia*

Laryngomalacia is by far the most commonly encountered reason for stridor in the neonate. Barthez and Riliet described the characteristic redundant, flaccid supraglottic laryngeal structures in 1853. The basic alterations that may be present are: 1.) an elongated and tubular epiglottis that collapses in on itself and posteriorly with inspiration, 2.) short aryepiglottic folds that collapse medially and 3.) bulky, redundant mucosa overlying the arytenoid cartilages that collapses anteriorly. There have been multiple theories put forward to explain the etiology of laryngomalacia, though lately, an underlying neurologic cause for laryngomalacia has become the most prominent.

Inspiratory stridor is the characteristic presenting complaint in laryngomalacia. Classically, the stridor increases in intensity with feeding, agitation, and supine positioning as opposed to prone. Stridor typically appears at birth or shortly thereafter, with an average of around 2 weeks [3], although in some cases, symptoms may not develop until several months of age [4, 5]. Symptoms worsen over the ensuing months, stabilize around 9 months of age, and begin to improve thereafter. Most infants will have resolution of their stridor by 18-24 months, although some patients (especially those with concomitant neurologic disease) may continue to be symptomatic for several years [5].

While laryngomalacia is most commonly mild enough to allow for conservative management, approximately 10-15% of patients will require surgical management. It is important to recognize the signs and symptoms separating a child with mild or moderate laryngomalacica from one with severe. Inspiratory stridor is a universal finding in children laryngomalacia, but children whose stridor is accompanied by respiratory compromise, hypoxia, or significant retractions are candidates for surgical intervention. Similarly, feeding difficulties are often seen in laryngomalacia patients. Commonly reported issues include: slow feeding, coughing, choking, and regurgitation. Children with severe laryngomalacia may present with failure to thrive, despite medical management.

A history of cyanotic or apparent life threatening apneic episodes is particularly concerning, and should spur a prompt workup and consideration for surgery. Finally, children with the serious sequelae of cor pulmonale and pulmonary hypertension should proceed to surgery.

Tracheotomy was the mainstay of surgical management for much of the 20<sup>th</sup> century. Supraglottoplasty is now the first-line operation for children with severe laryngomalacia. As described by Zalzal *et al.*, the operation consists of DSML followed by incising the aryepiglottic folds, releasing the epiglottis to spring forward, and trimming of the mucosa overlying the arytenoid and corniculate cartilages [1]. This is performed under general anesthesia ideally with the patient spontaneously breathing, although at times intubation is necessary, in which case the endotracheal tube can be briefly removed and excision performed while the child is apneic. Perioperative systemic steroids and inhaled racemic epinephrine can help to prevent troublesome post-operative laryngeal edema, and most children remain extubated after surgery.

Assisted breathing techniques (CPAP, BiPAP), or even tracheotomy should still be considered as options in patients with persistent severe symptoms following supraglottoplasty, or in patients whose comorbidities present other reasons for obtaining a surgical airway.

**Subglottic Stenosis**

Pathologic narrowing of the subglottis may be congenital, but is most often acquired, secondary to prolonged intubation. Congenital stenosis may involve any part of the larynx, most commonly the glottic and subglottic region, and may vary from a thin, membranous web, to a thick, long-segment stenosis. Likewise, acquired subglottic narrowing can vary in nature and degree. Obstruction may be caused by cysts arising from blocked mucus glands, granulation tissue, or thick, mature scar tissue. Subglottic stenosis is graded by severity, most commonly using the Cotton-Meyer scale [6]. According to this system, Grade I denotes an airway narrowed by less than 50%, Grade II from 51-70%, Grade III from 71-99%, and Grade IV indicates no discernible airway lumen.

Management for subglottic stenosis depends on multiple factors, including the location, severity, and type of narrowing present [7, 8]. In general, less severe

(Grades I and II) narrowing, and narrowing caused by a thin band or soft tissue can be successfully managed with endoscopic procedures. Severe stenoses, or those involving a long segment of the airway, or thick scar tissue require open procedures utilizing techniques such as cartilage grafting and airway resection and reanastomosis.

## Vocal Fold Paralysis

Vocal fold paralysis is another common cause of stridor in the neonate. Presentation, etiology, and management differs between unilateral paralysis and bilateral. Stridor is common to both groups of patients. Unilateral paralysis may also present with dysphonia (*i.e.* breathy voice, or weak cry) and feeding difficulty (including aspiration). Children with bilateral paralysis typically have a normal cry, but may present with respiratory distress. Diagnosis of vocal fold paralysis is best made with fiberoptic laryngoscopy in an awake patient.

Iatrogenic causes, specifically patent ductus arteriosus ligation and other cardiothoracic procedures predominate in unilateral paralysis. Bilateral paralysis is strongly associated with the Arnold-Chiari malformation. Other causes for paralysis, whether unilateral or bilateral include birth trauma, recent intubation, and a large group of patients for whom there is no readily identifiable cause [9].

A substantial number of children with vocal fold paralysis will recover function over time. Most of those who will recover do so within 2 years, though patients have been shown to recover function as far out as 11 years [10]. Patients with unilateral paralysis and no signs of aspiration should be observed until at least age 2 or 3 before any invasive treatments are pursued. Management of unilateral paralysis consists of techniques to medialize the affected cord in order to better approximate the healthy side during phonation, including injection with various short or long-lasting substances (*i.e.* collagen, micronized dermis, aqueous gel, fat, calcium hydroxyapetite), and open surgery utilizing implants to provide permanent medialization [11]. Bilateral paralysis may require tracheotomy initially if there is sufficient obstruction to cause respiratory distress. Further management is designed to lessen the obstruction to allow for decannulation, and includes both endoscopic and open techniques for vocal fold lateralization, removing a portion of one vocal fold and/or arytenoid cartilage, and using a costal cartilage graft with a posterior cricoid split.

## Recurrent Respiratory Papillomatosis

Recurrent respiratory papillomatosis (RRP) is caused by infection with the Human Papilloma Virus (HPV), most commonly subtypes 6 and 11 [12]. These are the same subtypes that cause genital condylomata. The virus leads to proliferation of benign squamous papillomas. Although rare, dysplasia and malignant transformation have been reported. Transmission occurs vertically. Greater than half of mothers of children with RRP had clinically evident genital condylomata at the time of delivery. Delivery by caesarean section seems to lower the rate of transmission, but is not routinely recommended.

Children with RRP most commonly present with hoarseness, but may be diagnosed after a progressive course of increasing respiratory compromise. Younger age at diagnosis correlates with more aggressive disease. Children diagnosed before age 3 are more than 3 times more likely to require more than 4 surgeries per year [13, 14]. The natural history is highly variable with some patients going into remission, while others progress to severe disease requiring frequent surgeries, or the fatal spread of disease into the distal airways.

Surgical debulking remains the mainstay of treatment. Numerous modalities have been used to accomplish this, including cold-steel excision, $CO_2$ laser, and microdebrider. Tracheotomy is reserved for only the most serious cases of airway obstruction, as this is strongly associated with development of tracheal papillomas. Multiple adjuvant therapies have been studied, including intralesional Cidofovir, interferon alpha-2a, indole-3-carbinol, among others.

## Subglottic Hemangioma

Infantile hemangiomas are the most common benign neoplasms in children. While rare, hemangiomas may present in the subglottis. Subglottic hemangiomas behave in the same manner as cutaneous lesions, with a proliferative phase starting 6-12 weeks post-natally and lasting about a year, followed by involution [15]. About 50% of children with a subglottic hemangioma will also have a cutaneous lesion.

Patients with hemangioma in a "beard" distribution on the face have an increased likelihood of subglottic hemangioma, as well as other abnormalities such as posterior fossa and cardiovascular anomalies (PHACES syndrome).

Depending on the size of the hemangioma, management can vary from medical management with systemic steroids, or more recently, oral Propranolol, to intralesional steroid injection, to excision ($CO_2$ laser *versus* open). Given its favorable side effect profile and excellent efficacy, Propranolol is more frequently being used as a first-line therapy. Multiple series have demonstrated its safety and efficacy in children with airway hemangiomas [16, 17]. Potential serious adverse effects with using Propranolol include hypotension and hypoglycemia, though these have been extremely rare in the reports to date.

### *Vascular Compression*

Several vascular anomalies have the potential to compress the airway [18]. Double aortic arch is the most common symptomatic anomaly. Others include pulmonary artery sling, aberrant right subclavian, and compression from the innominate artery. Diagnosis may be made by distinctive bronchoscopic findings and confirmed with either CT angiography or MRI.

### CONCLUSION

Stridor is a symptom that can arise from myriad causes. Successful management of the stridulous child requires a systematic approach to the history and physical exam.

### ACKNOWLEDGEMENT

Declared none.

### CONFLICT OF INTEREST

The authors confirm that this chapter content has no conflict of interest.

### REFERENCES

[1]     Zalzal GH, Anon JB, Cotton RT. Epiglottoplasty for the treatment of laryngomalacia. Ann Otol Rhinol Laryngol1987 Jan-Feb;96(1 Pt 1):72-6.

[2]     Zoumalan R, Maddalozzo J, Holinger LD. Etiology of stridor in infants. Ann Otol Rhinol Laryngol2007 May;116(5):329-34.

[3]     Olney DR, Greinwald JH, Jr., Smith RJ, Bauman NM. Laryngomalacia and its treatment. Laryngoscope1999 Nov;109(11):1770-5.

[4]     McSwiney PF, Cavanagh NP, Languth P. Outcome in congenital stridor (laryngomalacia). Arch Dis Child1977 Mar;52(3):215-8.

[5]     Smith GJ, Cooper DM. Laryngomalacia and inspiratory obstruction in later childhood. Arch Dis Child1981 May;56(5):345-9.

[6]     Myer CM, 3rd, O'Connor DM, Cotton RT. Proposed grading system for subglottic stenosis based on endotracheal tube sizes. Ann Otol Rhinol Laryngol1994 Apr;103(4 Pt 1):319-23.

[7]     Cotton RT. Management of subglottic stenosis. Otolaryngol Clin North Am2000 Feb;33(1):111-30.

[8]     Durden F, Sobol SE. Balloon laryngoplasty as a primary treatment for subglottic stenosis. Arch Otolaryngol Head Neck Surg2007 Aug;133(8):772-5.

[9]     Chen EY, Inglis AF, Jr. Bilateral vocal cord paralysis in children. Otolaryngol Clin North Am2008 Oct;41(5):889-901, viii.

[10]    Daya H, Hosni A, Bejar-Solar I, Evans JN, Bailey CM. Pediatric vocal fold paralysis: a long-term retrospective study. Arch Otolaryngol Head Neck Surg2000 Jan;126(1):21-5.

[11]    King EF, Blumin JH. Vocal cord paralysis in children. Curr Opin Otolaryngol Head Neck Surg2009 Dec;17(6):483-7.

[12]    Derkay CS, Wiatrak B. Recurrent respiratory papillomatosis: a review. Laryngoscope2008 Jul;118(7):1236-47.

[13]    Derkay CS. Task force on recurrent respiratory papillomas. A preliminary report. Arch Otolaryngol Head Neck Surg1995 Dec;121(12):1386-91.

[14]    Wiatrak BJ, Wiatrak DW, Broker TR, Lewis L. Recurrent respiratory papillomatosis: a longitudinal study comparing severity associated with human papilloma viral types 6 and 11 and other risk factors in a large pediatric population. Laryngoscope2004 Nov;114(11 Pt 2 Suppl 104):1-23.

[15]    TJ OL, Messner A. Subglottic hemangioma. Otolaryngol Clin North Am2008 Oct;41(5):903-11, viii-ix.

[16]    Truong MT, Perkins JA, Messner AH, Chang KW. Propranolol for the treatment of airway hemangiomas: a case series and treatment algorithm. Int J Pediatr Otorhinolaryngol Sep;74(9):1043-8.

[17]    Javia LR, Zur KB, Jacobs IN. Evolving treatments in the management of laryngotracheal hemangiomas: Will propranolol supplant steroids and surgery? International Journal of Pediatric Otorhinolaryngology;75(11):1450-4.

[18]    Berdon WE. Rings, slings, and other things: vascular compression of the infant trachea updated from the midcentury to the millennium--the legacy of Robert E. Gross, MD, and Edward B. D. Neuhauser, MD. Radiology2000 Sep;216(3):624-32.

*Send Orders of Reprints at reprints@benthamscience.net*

# CHAPTER 10

## Assessment and Management of Velopharyngeal Insufficiency

### Luke J. Schloegel[1] and Diego A. Preciado[2*]

*[1]Assistant Professor of Otolaryngology, Department of Otolaryngology, Kaiser Permanent Oakland, 3505 Broadway Oakland, CA 94611, USA and [2]Assistant Professor of Otolaryngology, Pediatrics, and Integrative Systems Biology, The George Washington University School of Medicine, Fellowship Program Director, Division of Pediatric Otolaryngology, Children's National Medical Center, Washington, DC, USA*

**Abstract:** The inability to communicate effectively can result in significant social-developmental compromise in children. Children who suffer from velopharyngeal insufficiency (VPI) will suffer from loss of volume and intelligibility of their speech, which is resultantly hypernasal.

Most causes of VPI in children are anatomic or neuromuscular. A history of cleft palate either before or after repair is the most common cause of VPI. The importance of syndrome recognition in patients with VPI is critical, as this population may be at particular risk for postoperative airway obstruction, respond less reliably to surgical correction, and require more aggressive adjunctive speech therapy.

The evaluation of VPI consists of a thorough history, physical examination, velopharyngeal assessment, and most importantly, a speech resonance analysis. A multidisciplinary approach consisting of an initial assessment conducted by an otolaryngologist and a speech pathologist is most effective for the diagnosis and management of VPI. Also, directed speech therapy remains a central component in the primary or adjunctive treatment of children with VPI.

In general, surgical procedures employed to treat VPI can be classified as palatal, palatopharyngeal, or pharyngeal. Outcomes after VPI surgery are probably dependent on a multitude of factors, including severity of preoperative VPI, gap size, presence or absence of comorbidities or syndromes and surgeon comfort.

**Keywords:** Velopharyngeal insufficiency, velopharyngeal dysfunction, cleft palate, submucous cleft palate, occult submucous cleft palate, hypernasal speech,

*****Address correspondence to Diego A. Preciado:** Assistant Professor of Otolaryngology, Pediatrics, and Integrative Systems Biology, The George Washington University School of Medicine, Fellowship Program Director, Division of Pediatric Otolaryngology, Children's National Medical Center, Washington, DC, USA; E-mail: dpreciad@cnmc.org

speech therapy, 22q11 deletion, perceptual speech evaluation, nasoendoscopy, sphincter pharyngoplasty, pharyngeal flap.

## INTRODUCTION

The ability to communicate through well-articulated speech is integral to being human and can have a large impact on the quality of one's life. Failure to produce intelligible speech can result in significant social developmental compromise in children, affecting a child's confidence and ability to integrate into groups. Proper articulation of speech requires coordination of a complex set of motor skills and anatomical integrity. It involves the production of an air column that travels from the lungs through the vocal cords and resonates out the oropharynx and oral cavity. Velopharyngeal closure is necessary for control of resonance in the oropharynx and ultimately the production of intelligible speech.

Velopharyngeal insufficiency (VPI) results from inadequate closure of the velopharyngeal sphincter during speech, which gives an abnormally hypernasal resonance to the voice. Occasionally, in severe cases, there may be nasal escape of swallowed foods as well. The production of all voiceless consonants except the nasal ones (m, n, and ng) requires high oral pressure. This is obtained when the soft palate seals off the oropharynx from the nasal cavity. If there is inadequate closure of the sphincter during speech, air escapes into the nose. VPI will alter the volume and intelligibility of speech to a varying degree depending on its severity and associated articulation disorders. Articulation errors, including compensatory misarticulation worsen the situation.

## ETIOLOGY

Most causes of velopharyngeal dysfunction in children are anatomic or neuromuscular. Anatomic causes may include history of cleft palate, submucous cleft palate, and history of adenoidectomy. Neuromuscular causes are related to impaired muscular control secondary to cerebral palsy or cardiovascular accident.

A history of cleft palate either before or after repair is the most common cause of velopharyngeal insufficiency. VPI has been reported in as many as 30-50% of patients following palate repair [1]. Studies have shown that children born with a complete cleft palate are more likely to require VPI surgery than compared to children with incomplete clefts [2].

Submucous cleft palate is a condition that is defined by the presence of a bifid uvula, a midline lucency of the soft palate, and notching of the hard palate. On the other hand, an occult submucosal cleft palate is a deficiency of the muscularis uvulae and diastasis of the levator veli palatini but without the presence of a bifid uvula or grooving of the oral surface of the soft palate. Most patients with either overt or occult submucous cleft palate can produce normal speech. However, because of their abnormal musculature, these patients may be predisposed to VPI from any changes to the velopharyngeal anatomy, such as adenoidectomy or velocardiofacial syndrome.

Transient VPI with hypernasal resonance following adenoidectomy, with or without tonsillectomy, is not uncommon. This condition may persist for several days to weeks and usually resolves spontaneously. Incidence of persistent VPI after adenoidectomy has been reported to be approximately 1 per 1,500 patients [3]. While the adenoid pad is not necessary for normal velopharyngeal closure, adenoidectomy can unmask a pre-existing palatal problem by removal of tissue against which a poorly functioning palate was achieving velopharyngeal closure. Children at risk of developing persistent VPI after adenoidectomy must be identified preoperatively by presence of repaired cleft palate, submucous cleft palate, 22q11 deletion, or neuromuscular problems. Speech therapy is first-line treatment for post-adenoidectomy VPI. Approximately 50% of post-adenoidectomy VPI children will require some form of surgical intervention [4].

Velopharyngeal insufficiency is seen in many syndromic children. A predisposition to VPI is seen in patients with trisomy 21. The combination of oromotor and developmental delays, generalized hypotonia, and intellectual delays constitute significant risk factors for development of VPI following adenoidectomy. Velocardiofacial syndrome (VCF) is an autosomal dominant entity linked to microdeletions in the long arm of chromosome 22. VPI has been reported to be present in approximately 75% of patients with 22q11 deletions, with only 10% of those patients showing actual submucous clefts, providing credence to the theory that VPI occurs in patients with either anatomic or syndromic, *i.e.* functional, causes [5]. Major findings in VCF include cleft palate (overt, submucous, or occult submucous), conotruncal heart anomalies, mental disabilities, and a characteristic facies. VPI is common in patients with VCF syndrome due to the presence of a cleft palate and pharyngeal hypotonia. The importance of syndrome recognition in patients with VPI is critical, as this population may be at particular risk for postoperative airway obstruction, respond less reliably to surgical correction, and require more aggressive adjunctive speech therapy [6].

Acquired VPI may present in persons affected by stroke or head injury, especially if damage occurs to motor centers controlling cranial nerves responsible for pharyngeal muscle control. Other neurologic diseases (*e.g.*, muscular dystrophy, multiple sclerosis, amyotrophic lateral sclerosis [ALS], Parkinson disease) also may lead to VPI in the more advanced stages of disease.

## ANATOMY

Six muscles comprise the velopharyngeal sphincter. Levator veli palatini is the major elevator of the soft palate. Its fibers fan out in the soft palate and blend with the contralateral levator. Innervated by the pharyngeal plexus from cranial nerve (CN) IX and X, contraction of this muscle moves the soft palate upward and backward into contact with the posterior pharyngeal wall. Abnormal insertion of the levator muscle is seen in overt and submucous cleft palate giving an anatomical basis for VPI in some cases. Tensor veli palatini arises from the scaphoid fossa, spine of the sphenoid, and the cartilaginous portion of the eustachian tube. It inserts into a tendon winding around the hamular process. Innervated by the mandibular branch of CN V, it tenses the soft palate and opens the eustachian tube during swallowing.

The Muscularis uvulae arises from the palatal aponeurosis posterior to the hard palate and inserts into the uvula mucosa. It functions to add bulk to the dorsal aspect of the uvula. Palatoglossus forms the anterior tonsillar pillar and simultaneously lowers the velum and elevates the tongue upwards and backwards. It depresses the palate for nasal speech. On the other hand, palatopharyngeus narrows the velopharyngeal orifice by adducting the posterior pillars and constricting the pharyngeal isthmus. The superior pharyngeal constrictor produces medial movement of the pharyngeal walls, narrowing the pharynx from side to side. The inferior portion of this muscle forms passavant's ridge. Early descriptions of speech described contact of the soft palate with this fold of the posterolateral pharyngeal wall. However, newer observations suggest that the soft palate contacts the posterior nasopharyngeal wall above the level of this ridge [7].

## EVALUATION

The evaluation of VPI consists of a thorough history, physical examination, velopharyngeal assessment, and most importantly, a speech resonance analysis. A multidisciplinary approach consisting of an initial assessment conducted by an otolaryngologist and a speech pathologist is most effective for the diagnosis and management of VPI. Also, directed speech therapy remains a central component in the primary or adjunctive treatment of children with VPI.

Patient history can provide important information concerning the diagnosis of VPI. The history should include pertinent questions about perinatal difficulties, previous diagnosis of cleft palate, and other co-morbidities, which may indicate the presence of a congenital syndrome. Parents should also be questioned about symptoms consistent with sleep apnea, snoring, or otitis media. Hearing loss can interfere with language acquisition, and hearing in patients with VPI should be evaluated early and regularly. In patients suspected of having obstructive sleep apnea, a polysomnography is indicated. Children with both obstructive sleep apnea and VPI should have treatment of the sleep apnea prior to surgical management of VPI [8]. Finally, exploring the social impact of the child's speech intelligibility can affect management strategies. Children with significant social integration issues may warrant more aggressive treatment.

A thorough physical examination is critical in the evaluation of children with VPI. Otoscopy allows examination of the tympanic membrane for findings that may indicate eustachian tube dysfunction. All clinicians should be aware of the increased risk for conductive hearing loss in patients with VPI and diagnose chronic serous otitis media appropriately. Examination of the anterior nose is used to assess the septum and mucosa. Importantly, the oropharyngeal examination will reveal abnormalities of the palate, uvula, and tonsils. Enlarged tonsils, themselves, may affect palatal elevation and contribute to VPI. Occasionally, tonsillectomy with cephalad adenoidectomy, may have a favorable effect on VPI [8].

If velopharyngeal insufficiency is suspected in a child, physical assessment of velopharyngeal sphincter closure and function is performed by nasoendosocpy, or by radiographic multiview video fluoroscopy (MVF), or by both. Nasoendoscopy allows the physician to directly visualize velopharyngeal closure during speech and estimate the size of the gap. Velopharyngeal closure patterns are described as coronal, circular or sagittal. Furthermore, it allows the surgeon to characterize the mobility in order to tailor the surgical procedure to the defect. Patients with poor anterior-posterior motion and good lateral wall motion are reportedly better suited to undergo a pharyngeal flap. On the other hand, patients with poorer lateral wall motion but some intact anterior-posterior palatal motion should undergo sphincter pharyngoplasty. The examination is recorded and can be easily shared among clinicians; also pre- and post-operative comparisons can be made. Studies have demonstrated fairly good interrater reliability with the usage of nasoendoscopy to assess VPI,[9] and nasoendosocpy has been shown to correlate better with VPI severity than MVF [10].

For MVF, barium instilled through the nose coats the surface of the velum and posterior pharyngeal wall, allowing visualization of these structures. Lateral, anterior/posterior, and base views are required to obtain true measurements of the velopharyngeal sphincter. However, difficulties with overlapping shadows, positioning, and asymmetry can make the interpretation of MVF difficult [11]. Concerns with radiation dosages have tempered the enthusiasm for MVF in many centers. Many centers have abandoned the usage of MVF, relying on nasoendoscopy alone [11]. Recently, there have been reports in the literature of the use of magnetic resonance (MR) imaging to assess VPI. MR data may have a place in assessing the palate muscle size, distribution, and position, but it should not be used as a front-line diagnostic procedure for assessing VPI [12].

Perceptual speech evaluation is also performed by a speech-language pathologist and is of central importance in the diagnosis of VPI and predicting postsurgical outcomes. This evaluation examines all aspects of speech production, including voice, articulation, oral motor sequencing, and velopharyngeal function. It is important to distinguish velopharyngeal mislearning from VPI as mislearning is the result of articulation problems and may respond to speech therapy alone.

As an initial step in the subjective assessment, the examining clinical team should focus on the voiceless consonants such as p, t, k, s, f, and sh which require maximal pulmonary pressures and thus can be used as a good screening measure for integrity of plosive sounds. Phonemes that require VP closure such as 'sk', 'six', 'sp', or 'pt' should also be elicited. Having the child count from sixty to sixty-six will often elicit abnormal speech patterns. Finally overall intelligibility in running, spontaneous, connected speech should also be ascertained. This assessment of perceptual speech has been shown to be useful in predicting relative velopharyngeal gap size [13]. The Pittsburg Weighted Speech Scale is used in many clinics to report severity of VPI in a semi-objective fashion that is comparable pre- and postoperatively and among centers [14].

Objective tools for assessment of hypernasality also exist. Nasalance, a measure of hypernasality, can be determined by a nasometer, a tool that can evaluate the ratio of nasal to oral air emission during speech [15]. Although results from nasometry are compared to normalized values for standard speech passages, they do not correlate well with the size of the velopharyngeal gap and do not correlate well with treatment outcomes for VPI [8]. High nasometry ratio scores are generated when there is increased nasal air emission. However, a small velopharyngeal gap may often release a paradoxically high steam of airflow pressure, making an audible noise and generating a misleadingly high nasalance score. Therefore, the clinical interpretation of the nasometry score needs to be done properly and in the context of the subjective speech perception assessment. Aerodynamic measurements of absolute nasal airflow in cc/sec can a useful adjunct in the objective assessment of VPI, [16] but have not been as universally used in most treatment centers. As with nasometry, airflow data do not provide information on the size of location of the velopharyngeal gap in patients with VPI.

## MANAGEMENT

The treatment of VPI begins with directed speech therapy to correct compensatory misarticulations. Early speech therapy results in increased speech accuracy and can help improve long-term outcomes. Parents can be trained to effectively deliver speech therapy to young children with cleft palate [17]. Surgery is proposed when continued speech therapy no longer improves the patient's speech. It is important to note that some speech therapists employ "oral-motor therapy" such as blowing, sucking massage, *etc.* These techniques have never been demonstrated to be of any value and all clinicians should make sure that their patients are not receiving ineffective speech therapy [18].

The use of prosthetic appliances can be a conservative option for intervention in VPI. Common prosthetic appliances include palatopharyngeal obturators, palatal lifts, or pharyngeal bulbs. Prosthetic management is often employed in children who are poor surgical candidates. They can improve velopharyngeal dysfunction but compliance can be an issue in children who refuse to wear them [19].

Surgical intervention is probably the most popular treatment methodology because outcomes are generally good and patient compliance is not required. There has been a movement toward tailoring the choice of surgical procedure employed to the specific defect noted in the patient [20]. Some claim that successful outcomes in fact depend on matching the functional capability of the patient with the surgical procedure. Others have disputed this claim reporting that there is no difference in outcome regardless of surgical technique or preoperative sphincter characteristics [21].

In general, surgical procedures employed to treat VPI can be classified as palatal, palatopharyngeal, or pharyngeal. Palatal procedures most often include the Furlow palatoplasty, which involves a double Z-plasty lengthening of the palate [22]. This technique appears to work best when the orientation of the palatal levator musculature is sagittal[8] or when a small preoperative velopharyngeal gap size is noted [23].

The most common palatopharyngeal technique employed is the superiorly based pharyngeal flap. This procedure involves the creation of a superiorly based myomucosal flap from the pharyngeal wall that is inserted into the nasal surface of the soft palate, creating two lateral pharyngeal ports. It is best utilized when there is severe hypernasality in the setting of a large central velopharyngeal gap and good lateral wall movement [8]. The drawback to this surgery is the potential for prolonged postoperative obstructive sleep apnea (OSA) development in up to 50% of patients [24]. Care must be taken in the pediatric population to ensure the adequacy of nasal respiration following pharyngeal flap surgery. In many cases, this includes hyper vigilance for OSA both before and after surgery. Surgeons should definitely contemplate removal of large tonsils and adenoids prior to pharyngeal flap surgery.

At times the pharyngeal flap procedure seems excessive compared to the size of the velopharyngeal (VP) defect. Pharyngeal procedures for VPI treatment include augmentation of the posterior pharyngeal wall and sphincter pharyngoplasty. Augmentation pharyngoplasty is contemplated when VPI is mild and characterized by a small coronal gap. However results of rolled muscle flaps to augment the coronal gap and pharynx have not been encouraging [25]. The sphincter palatoplasty consists of raising two myomucosal flaps of the posterior pharyngeal wall just superior to the level of the velum. Theoretically, the sphincter becomes dynamic. However, one study featured selective electromyographic evaluation of the muscular pharyngeal sphincter during speech and revealed no intrinsic muscular activity. It is important to place these flaps high in the sphincter to reduce the need for revision surgery [26]. The sphincter pharyngoplasty has also been recommended for use in cases of stress-induced VPI, such as in wind instrument players [27].

Injectable and implantable materials can be used to augment the posterior pharyngeal wall when the VP gap is small. Infectious complications, granuloma formation, migration, or resorption have been associated with many of these injectable materials, including silastic, proplast, cartilage, Teflon, and collagen. Recent reports of injectable hydroxyapatite hold promise for mild VPI treatment, but are outside of the Food and Drug Administration (FDA) recommendations [28].

## OUTCOMES

Complications after VPI surgery include persistent VPI, flap dehiscence, and OSA. Concerns about long-term OSA development after pharyngeal flap surgery have led some centers to abandon its usage all together [29]. A recent study with a large sample size of 222 consecutive pharyngeal flap operations reported a relatively low postoperative OSA incidence and concluded that when appropriately performed, pharyngeal flap surgery was a well tolerated and effective operation for the treatment of VPI, and that was no reason to avoid applying it to children for fears of post-operative OSA [30]. In the case of severe persistent OSA after superiorly based pharyngeal flap, division of the flap generally results in improvement in symptoms and some persistent speech benefit.

Perceptual speech assessment is a key subjective tool used to diagnose VPI in children, determine disease severity, and measure improvement after treatment. Speech intelligibility is very important to patients with VPI and can have a large impact on quality of life. Both the trained ear of the otolaryngologist and speech pathologist and that of the lay public can be one of the best methods of understanding outcomes in patients who undergo VPI surgery. It is also important to develop standardized methods for use in research and improve overall management of patients with VPI. One study validated a new disease-specific instrument, the Velopharyngeal Insufficiency Quality of Life (VPIQL) survey. This study identified that children with VPI and their parents perceive a reduced quality of life when compared with age-matched controls [31]. Another prospective cohort study implemented the Pediatric Voice Outcome Survey, an instrument used to assess general voice-related quality of life, and showed that parents perceived at least short-term improvements in functional outcomes and quality of life following surgery for VPI in their children [32].

The greatest predictor for postoperative final speech outcomes from VPI surgery is the preoperative condition of the patient. Children with syndromes, such as velocardiofacial, as compared to those with anatomic, non-syndromic causes of VPI are more likely to have suboptimal outcomes after surgery [6,25,33]. The type of surgical procedure employed does not seem to be as important as the experience of the surgeon. A large, prospective, randomized study from Spain found no difference in outcomes when comparing sphincter pharyngoplasty to pharyngeal flaps, regardless of the preoperative VP sphincter characteristics [21]. In summary, outcomes after VPI surgery are probably dependent on a multitude of factors, including severity of preoperative VPI, gap size, presence or absence of comorbidities or syndromes and surgeon comfort.

There seems to be no long-term effect on growth after VP closure over time. The ratio of cephalometric measurements of velar length to pharyngeal depth was similar in patients with repaired clefts and their normal control subjects. This ratio remained stable with growth from 4 years of age through puberty [34].

## CONCLUSION

The evaluation and management of VPI require a coordinated multidisciplinary approach by a group of providers familiar with the anatomy and function of the VP sphincter. Current reports show that outcomes and complications are comparable for Furlow palatoplasty, pharyngeal flap, and sphincter pharyngoplasty. Research and standardization of evaluation techniques are needed to better compare outcomes across treatment centers to optimize treatment strategies.

## ACKNOWLEDGEMENT

Declared none.

## CONFLICT OF INTEREST

The authors have no financial conflicts of interest to disclose.

## REFERENCES

[1]     de Buys Roessingh AS, Cherpillod J, *et al.* Speech outcome after cranial-based pharyngeal flap in children born with total cleft, cleft palate, or primary velopharyngeal insufficiency. *J Oral Maxillofac Surg.* Dec 2006;64(12):1736-42.
[2]     McWilliams BJ, Morris HL, Shelton RJ: Cleft Palate Speech. Philadelphia: BC Decker, 1990.
[3]     Witzel MA, Rich RH, Margar-Bacal F, Cox C. Velopharyngeal insufficiency after adenoidectomy: an 8-year review. *Int J Pediatr Otorhinolaryngol.* Feb 1986;11(1):15-20.
[4]     Saunders NC, Hartley BE, Sell D, Sommerlad B. Velopharyngeal insufficiency following adenoidectomy. *Clin Otolaryngol Allied Sci.* Dec 2004; 29 (6): 686-8.
[5]     Dyce O, McDonal-McGinn D, Kirschner RE, *et al.* Otolaryngologic manifestations of the 22q11.2 deletion syndrome. *Arch Otolaryngol Head Neck Surg* 2002; 128:1408-12.
[6]     Losken A, Williams JK, Burstein FD, *et al.* Surgical correction of velopharyngeal insufficiency in children with velocardiofacial syndrome. *Plast Reconstr Surg* 2006; 117: 1493-8.
[7]     Janfaza P, Nadol JB, *et al. Surgical Anatomy of the Head and Neck.* Boston: Harvard University Press, 2011.

[8]     Rudnick EF, Sie KC. Velopharyngeal insufficiency: current concepts in diagnosis and management. Curr Opin Otolaryng Head Neck Surg. Dec 2008;16(6):530-5.

[9]     Sie KC, Starr JR, Bloom DC, Cunningham M, de Serres LM, Drake AF, *et al.* Multicenter interrater and intrarater reliability in the endoscopic evaluation of velopharyngeal insufficiency. Arch Otolaryngol Head Neck Surg. Jul 2008;134(7):757-63

[10]    Lam DJ, Starr JR, Perkins JA, *et al.* A comparison of nasoendoscopy and multiview videofluoroscopy in assessing velopharyngeal insufficiency. *Otolaryngol Head Neck Surg* 2006; 134: 394-402.

[11]    Willging JP. Velopharyngeal Insufficiency. *Curr Opin Otolaryngol Head Neck Surg*. Dec 2003; 11(6): 452-5.

[12]    Shprintzen RJ, Marrinan E. Velopharyngeal insufficienc: diagnosis and management. *Curr Opin Otolaryngol Head Neck Surg* 2009; 17: 302-7.

[13]    Kummer AW, Briggs M, Lee L. The relationship between the characteristics of speech and velopharyngeal gap size. *Cleft Palate Craniofac J* 2003; 40:590-96.

[14]    Dudas JR, Deleyiannis FW, Ford MD, *et al.* Diagnosis and treatment of velopharyngeal insufficiency: clinical utility of speech evaluation and video-fluoroscopy. *Ann Plast Surg* 2006; 56:511-517.

[15]    Hardin MA, Van Demark DR, Morris HL, Payne MM. Correspondence between nasalance scores and listener judgments of hypernasality and hyponasality. *Cleft Palate Craniofac J* 1992; 29:346-51.

[16]    Dotevall H, Lohmander-Agerskov A, Ejnell H, Bake B. Perceptual evaluation of speech and velopharyngeal function in children with without cleft palate and the relationship to nasal airflow patterns. *Cleft Palate Craniofac J* 2002; 39:409-24.

[17]    Scherer NJ, D'Antonio LL, McGahey H. Early intervention for speech impairment in children with cleft palate. *Cleft Palate Craniofac J* 2008;45:18-31.

[18]    Ruscello DM. An examination of nonspeech oral motor exercises for children with velopharyngeal inadequacy. *Semin Speech Lang* 2008; 29:294-303.

[19]    Pinto JH, da Silva DG, Pegoraro-Krook MI. Speech intelligibility of patients with cleft lip and palate after placement of speech prosthesis. *Cleft Palate Craniofac J* 2007; 44: 635-41.

[20]    Dixon-Wood VL, Williams WN, Seagle MB. Team acceptance of specific recommendations for the treatment of VPI provided by speech pathologists. *Cleft Palate Craniofac J* 1991; 28: 285-90; discussion 290-2.

[21]    Ysunza A, Pamplona C, Ramírez E, Molina F, Mendoza M, Silva A. Velopharyngeal surgery: a prospective randomized study of pharyngeal flaps and sphincter pharyngoplasties. Plast Reconstr Surg. Nov 2002;110(6):1401-7.

[22]    Furlow LT, Jr. Cleft palate repair by double opposing Z-plasty. *Plast Reconstr Surg* 1986; 78:724-38.

[23]    Dailey SA, Karnell MP, Karnell LH, Canady JW. Comparison of resonance outcomes after pharyngeal flap and Furlow double-opposing z-plasty for surgical management of velopharyngeal incompetence. *Cleft Palate Craniofac J* 2006; 43:38-43.

[24]    Liao YF, Chuang ML, Chen PK, *et al.* Incidence and severity of obstructive sleep apnea following pharyngeal flap surgery in patients with cleft palate. *Cleft Palate Craniofac J* 2002; 39:312-6.

[25]    Witt PD, O'Daniel TG, Marsh JL, Grames LM, Muntz HR, Pilgram TK. Surgical management of velopharyngeal dysfunction: outcome analysis of autogenous posterior pharyngeal wall augmentation. Plast Reconstr Surg. Apr 1997;99(5):1287-96; discussion 1297-300.

[26] Pryor LS, Lehman J, Parker MG, Schmidt A, Fox L, Murthy AS. Outcomes in pharyngoplasty: a 10-year experience. Cleft Palate Craniofac J. Mar 2006;43(2):222-5.

[27] McVicar R, Edmonds J, Kearns D. Sphincter pharyngoplasty for correction of stress velopharyngeal insufficiency. Otolaryngol Head Neck Surg 2002; 127:248-50.

[28] Sipp JA, Ashland J, Hartnick CJ. Injection pharyngoplasty with calcium hydroxyapatite for treatment of velopalatal insufficiency. Arch Otolaryngol Head Neck Surg. Mar 2008;134(3):268-71.

[29] Kravath RE, Pollak CP, Borowiecki B, Weitzman ED. Obstructive sleep apnea and death associated with surgical correction of velopharyngeal incompetence. *J Pediatr* 1980; 96:645-8.

[30] Cole P, Banerji S, Hollier L, Stal S. Two hundred twenty-two consecutive pharyngeal flaps: an analysis of postoperative complications. J Oral Maxillofac Surg. Apr 2008;66(4):745-8.

[31] Barr L, Thibeault SL, Muntz H, de Serres L. Quality of life in children with velopharyngeal insufficiency. Arch Otolaryngol Head Neck Surg. Mar 2007;133(3):224-9

[32] Boseley ME, Hartnick CJ. Assessing the outcome of surgery to correct velopharyngeal insufficiency with the pediatric voice outcomes survey. Int J Pediatr Otorhinolaryngol. Nov 2004;68(11):1429-33.

[33] Persson C, Elander A, Lohmander-Agerskov A, Soderpalm E. Speech outcomes in isolated cleft palate: impact of cleft extent and additional malformations. *Cleft Palate Craniofac J* 2002; 39:397-408.

[34] Satoh K, Wada T, Tachimura T, Shiba R. The effect of growth of nasopharyngeal structures in velopharyngeal closure in patients with repaired cleft palate and controls without clefts: a cephalometric study. Br J Oral Maxillofac Surg. Apr 2002;40(2):105-9.

Send Orders of Reprints at reprints@benthamscience.net

# CHAPTER 11

# Update on Recurrent Respiratory Papilloma – Current Thoughts and Management

## Craig Derkay[1]* and Michael DeMarcantonio[2]

*[1]Children's Hospital of the King's Daughters, Eastern Virginia Medical School, Norfolk, Virginia, USA and [2]Eastern Virginia Medical School, Norfolk, Virginia, USA*

**Abstract:** Recurrent respiratory papilloma is a disease process that has significant implications for the patient as well as socioeconomic implications as the disease is costly both in individual and societal terms. The pediatrician plays an essential role in both the diagnosis and management of children with RRP. Only through thorough knowledge and astute observation can delay in diagnosis be avoided, appropriate referral initiated, and suffering of this disease alleviated.

**Keywords:** RRP, human papilloma virus, HPV, cidofivir, interferon, gardisel.

## INTRODUCTION

Hoarseness is a common presenting complaint in the pediatrician's office. During childhood 4-23% of all children will present with hoarseness [1-3]. A majority of patients will manifest a short course with spontaneous resolution. These patients will be diagnosed with common conditions such as upper respiratory tract illnesses, laryngitis and gastro-esophageal reflux disease. It is crucial, however, to remember that in the pediatric population the second most common cause of hoarseness is Recurrent Respiratory Papillomatosis (RRP) [4]. Unlike the more common diseases mentioned above RRP is a serious condition that imparts severe morbidity and occasionally mortality.

RRP is a disease of the upper airway of viral etiology. Grossly this disease presents with benign exophytic lesions with a propensity for the supraglottis, glottis and trachea (Fig. **1**). The use of the word "benign" can be misleading in the

*Address correspondence to Craig Derkay:** Children's Hospital of the King's Daughters, Eastern Virginia Medical School, Norfolk, Virginia, USA; Tel: 757-668-9853; Fax: 757-668-9329; E-mail: derkaycs@evms.edu

discussion of RRP. Lesions warrant this classification due to their non-malignant pathology and a risk of malignant transformation of only 1-5% [5]. In spite of this classification, RRP imparts significant morbidity. Patients will often experience voice changes, progressive stridor and in some cases near complete airway obstruction. The disease is notorious for its mercurial course with some patient's experiencing spontaneous resolution and others a long protracted and progressive decline. The incidence of a RRP ranges from 1.7 to 4.3 cases per 100,000, making it relatively rare in the same range as Kawasaki's disease and pediatric brain tumors [6,7]. Despite its rarity the costs of the disease are great in both a personal and economic sense. The diagnosis and eventual treatment of these patients involves a large multi-disciplined treatment team frequently including pediatricians, otolaryngologists, clinical researchers and social workers. It is crucial for the pediatrician to understand the etiology, presentation and treatment of this disorder to allow for timely referral and diagnosis as well as continued surveillance and family support.

## Classification

Presentation of RRP can occur at nearly any age with patients being diagnosed prior to their 1st birthday and as late as after their 80th. Age of diagnosis is used to classify patients into two categories. Patient's presenting prior to 12 years of is classified as juvenile onset recurrent respiratory papillomatosis (JORRP). Those patients presenting at or after their 12th birthday are labeled as adult onset recurrent respiratory papillomatosis (AORRP). JORRP patients generally are diagnosed between the ages of 2 to 4, with 75% of patients being diagnosed before the age of 5 [8]. Despite this relatively early age of diagnosis, most patients experience an average delay of diagnosis of 1-2 years [9-10]. Boys and girls appear to be equally affected by JORRP [11]. With regards to predictors of severity, age of diagnosis is associated with more severe course. This finding is not surprising given that patient's diagnosed at an earlier age likely have severe symptoms that could not be confused with milder and more common entities.

In comparison, AORRP patients have a slight male predilection with a peak incidence of presentation between 20 and 40 years of age [12]. It should be noted that some patients will straddle these two classification groups. These patients, a subset of JORRP, will be diagnosed in childhood and have progressive disease into adulthood. This group can be classified as juvenile onset disease with persistence into adulthood.

## Etiology

The causative agent in RRP remained elusive until recently. The viral agent Human Papilloma Virus (HPV) had long been a prime suspect but only with the development of viral DNA probes could suspicions be confirmed. HPV is a small DNA containing, non-enveloped icosahedral capsid with double stranded DNA. Typically, HPV is associated with condylomata acuminata of the anus, vulva, penis and cervix. There are currently 100 serotypes of HPV identified. All serotypes are not created equally, with HPV 16,18,31 and 33 most commonly associated with malignant transformation. In the setting of RRP, HPV 6 and 11 have been associated with a majority of cases with other serotypes such as HPV 16 and 18 occasionally identified [13].

## Transmission

While the causative agent has been isolated and identified the method of transmission remains elusive. What is certain is that HPV is a ubiquitous infection. Ten percent of women of child bearing age will demonstrate active DNA positive disease while 60% show HPV antibodies reflecting previous infection [14]. In addition 1.5-5% of pregnant women will be diagnosed with an active HPV infection [14]. With these findings it seems reasonable to propose that vertical transmission from mother to child is a likely form of transmission [15-17]. To support this theory it has been demonstrated that children born to a mother with active condyloma are at 231 fold increased risk of developed [18]. Other researchers have found that 54% of patient with JORRP were born to mothers with vulvar condyloma at the time of delivery [19]. While this evidence appears to support vertical transmission it must be acknowledged that a majority of children born to women with condyloma do not develop RRP. This fact points to a more complex transmission process than simply direct exposure. Attempts have been made to isolate specific risk factors for transmission. Vaginal delivery, labor > 10 hours and being a first-born child, have been shown to increase transmission [18, 20]. It is proposed that these scenarios all present opportunities for prolonged labor and consequently prolonged exposure.

## Epidemiology

The incidence of RRP has been a subject of significant research in both the United States and abroad. In the United States incidence has been estimated to range from 1.7 to 4.3 cases per 100,000 in children and 1.8 cases per 100,000 in adults [6,11]. In a particularly thorough Danish study 50% of the population was surveyed revealing an incidence of 3.63 cases per 100,000 [21]. In contrast, Campisi and colleagues estimated incidence and prevalence using a patient registry. Their efforts resulted in an incidence of 0.24 per 100,000 and a prevalence of 1.11 per 100,000 [22]. This discrepancy is thought to be as a result of data extrapolation or an inherent variability in geographic incidence. Some efforts to explain this variability have focused on socio-economic status. At Toronto's sick Children's Hospital Leung *et al.* reported that half of patients with RRP were below the poverty line [18]. Within the U.S., Marisco and colleagues have shown that there is a variance in RRP incidence based on the type of hospital evaluated. In private hospitals, incidence is found to be 1.98 per 100,000 compared to 3.21 per 100,000 in public hospitals [17]. It has been suggested that this finding is a reflection of public hospitals treating a large number of lower socioeconomic patients. It must be remembered that "public" hospital would include academic institutions perhaps reflecting a selection/referral bias. Clearly, more research is needed to further define incidence and the factors that increase the risk of RRP development.

## Disease Course

The course of RRP is quite variable ranging from spontaneous resolution to unrelenting progression. Generally JORRP patients will require early and frequent surgical interventions. One study of Academic Pediatric Otolaryngology centers found that children with RRP averaged 19.7 surgeries with 4.4 surgeries per year [11]. Certain risk factors have been associated with a more aggressive course. These include younger age at diagnosis and HPV 11 serotype [13]. Patients with HPV 11 disease were found to require more frequent operative intervention, more frequent adjuvant therapy and be more likely to develop tracheal disease [13]. As with any benign neoplastic disease there remains a concern for malignant transformation. Fortunately, in the pediatric population the prevalence of dysplasia is only 1%. In comparison, in the setting of AORRP dysplasia can be found in 22 to 55% of patients. Overall the risk of malignant transformation is low ranging form 1-5% [5]. The greatest risk for mortality from RRP is associated with severe airway obstruction and extra-laryngeal spread. Children less than 2 years of age can present with severe airway obstruction and airway compromise resulting in death. More chronically, 10-13% of children will demonstrate progressive disease with extralaryngeal spread [6]. The most common sites involved include the oral cavity, trachea and bronchi. Those patients experiencing pulmonary spread frequently develop particularly progressive and destructive disease.

## CLINICAL FEATURES

### Presentation and History

Patients with RRP can present anytime during childhood but generally present as toddlers or pre-school age children. Hoarseness is the most common symptom at presentation. In infants prior to speech development, hoarseness may be relayed as a harsh or raspy cry. As discussed previously, hoarseness can be a non-specific and often innocuous symptom. Parental history is crucial to further elucidating the cause of the hoarseness. Questioning must focus on history of prematurity, airway truama, intubation, and maternal HPV infection. The course of the child's hoarseness and accompanying symptoms can be useful in determining the need for further workup. In particular, primary care physicians should be alert for hoarseness that fails to resolve or becomes progressive in nature, as this may be a harbinger of RRP. In addition, some patients will present with the clinical triad of hoarseness, stridor and airway obstruction. It must be remembered that when airway symptoms are present the patient must undergo an initial and rapid evaluation for safety. Any patient with obvious respiratory distress should be urgently medically transported to the nearest Emergency Department.

### Physical Exam

If stable the primary physician may proceed with physical examination. Observation of the patient's respirations should focus on retractions of abdomen/chest and flaring of nasal ala. Auscultation should attempt to differentiate stertor from stridor. Stertor is defined as a coarse snoring noise produced as a result of obstruction above the level of the larynx. Stridor in comparison is a high pitched whistling noise with inspiration, expiration or both phases and often associated with supraglottic, glottic or subglottic narrowing. The location of the lesion can often be deduced by the phase of respiration in which stridor occurs. Inspiratory stridor is associated with supraglottic lesions while expiratory stridor is associated with pulmonary or tracheal disease. Biphasic stridor often heralds a lesion at the level of the true vocal folds. In the setting of RRP stridor may progress from inspiratory to biphasic as undiagnosed disease progresses. It is important to attempt to distinguish inspiratory stridor caused by laryngomalacia from a more severe disease process. Generally patients with laryngomalacia will present with stridor that is worsened with position and activity. These patients inspiratory stridor is worsened by supine position, feeding and agitation. While RRP and other airway lesions such as subglottic stenosis will not vary and may be progressive in nature.

**Referral and Airway Endoscopy**

Pediatricians should consider referral for Otolaryngology evaluation in the following settings:

1.  Persistent or progressively worsening hoarseness.

2.  Hoarseness accompanied by stridor.

3.  Symptoms requiring emergency room evaluation for airway compromise.

Evaluation by an otolaryngologist will include the standard physical examination with the addition of airway endoscopy. In a stable patient <1 year of age or older than 6 years of age, an office flexible fiberoptic laryngoscopy (FFL) can be attempted to evaluate the supraglottis and glottis. This exam confirms true vocal fold mobility and can identify gross papilloma disease. Patients who can not tolerate flexible exam, those with gross disease and those with a normal FFL but high suspicion of RRP will need operative airway endoscopy.

Operative endoscopy includes awake flexible fiberoptic laryngoscopy, direct laryngoscopy, and rigid bronchsocopy. The abbreviation DLB will often be used to signify direct laryngoscopy and bronchoscopy. This operative examination will occur is systematic fashion examining all aspects of the larynx and trachea. Typically lesions will be found at junctional sites in the airway [23]. At these sites ciliated columnar mucosa transitions to squamous epithelium. Examples of these junction sites include the false cords, ventricles and undersurface of the true vocal cords. Examination of the trachea is important as the diagnosis of tracheal disease may indicate a more aggressive course. An interesting discrepancy between severity of symptoms and operative findings has been noted over the years. Clinical symptoms are remarkably dependent on specific anatomic location rather than bulk of disease. As an example a large supraglottic papilloma may be relatively asymptomatic while a very small lesion at the anterior junction of the true vocal folds could cause severe hoarseness and airway obstruction. This discrepancy highlights the need for operative endoscopy.

## Staging

Many differing staging systems have been proposed to quantify the severity and burden of RRP. Such a system is necessary for several reasons. The subjective nature of RRP symptoms and its variable course require an objective way to measure disease response to treatment. In addition a well-designed standardize staging system allows for easy communication between surgeons and standardization for research. In 1998 the RRP task force developed a staging system referred to as the Derkay-Coltera RRP staging system [24]. The scoring system combines subjective and objective measures. The subjects voice, stridor and airway status are first assigned a score. This score is then combined with anatomic staging score. For this score the subsites of the airway are assigned a score from 0 to 3, with 0=No lesion, 1= surface lesion, 2=raised lesion, 3= bulky lesion (Fig. **2**). This system allows for standardization of staging for easy communication between specialists, researchers and primary care physicians. It has demonstrated high reliability, low variance and most importantly a high level of surgeon-to-surgeon reliability [25]. In addition software designed by the University of Washington (Seattle) is now computerized and available for otolaryngologists to track an individual patients disease course and response to therapy.

# TREATMENT

## Surgical Therapy

Surgical therapy is the mainstay treatment in RRP. The goal of such therapy is to reduce tumor burden, decrease spread of disease, improve voice quality, and increase the interval between surgical procedures. However, all of these goals are secondary to maintaining an airway and doing no harm to the patient. As a result, aggressive removal of disease must often be forsaken and residual disease left to avoid damaging mucosa and creating scarring. Such airway scarring if created could prove to be irreversible and leave the patient with a worse airway than prior to intervention. As often stated, disease course and severity are quite variable. As a result, the need for surgical intervention varies form patient to patient and may fluctuate for an individual patient. At tertiary children's hospital's 50% of patients will require 10 procedures to control their disease while 7% of patient will need an astonishing 100 or more procedures throughout their lifetime [6]. Generally, patients diagnosed earlier in life will require more operative intervention. Patients diagnosed before age 3 are 3.6 times more likely to need to need >4 surgical procedures and 2.1 times more likely to have two anatomic sites involved, than children diagnosed a later age [11].

## Surgical Techniques

Many surgical techniques have been advocated for the treatment of RRP with frequent shifts in surgeon preference. Initially, cold steel excision was the only available technique. Today, however, microdebrider and $CO_2$ laser excision techniques have emerged as the two most common forms of therapy. Cold steel continues to be advocated primarily in the adult setting. Zeitels and Sataloff have shown acceptable recurrence rates in this population with low rates of complication and scar formation [26]. After its introduction, $CO_2$ laser became the primary mode of treatment. This therapy uses an invisible spectrum 10,600 nm laser in combination with a microscope to reduce disease burden. In contrast the microdebrider uses a protected oscillating blade coupled with suction to remove papilloma. A similar instrument has been used for years in sinus surgery and for adenoidectomy. Microdebrider has been purported to have several advantages over $CO_2$ laser excision. In comparing the two modalities microdebrider has been shown to have equivocal pain scores, improved voice outcomes, shorter procedure time and lower cost [27]. Objectively voice outcomes have also been shown to be superior in the immediate and early postoperative period [28]. Perhaps a result of these findings in a survey of pediatric otolaryngologists there has been a shift from cold steel and $CO_2$ laser to the use of microdebrider. It should be noted that all comparison studies to date are small and relatively short sighted in terms of follow-up. In addition removal of disease burden can effectively be completed safely with either technique in skilled hands. As a result both therapies remain standard of care. Unfortunately, in cases of recalcitrant disease or airway obstruction at presentation, a tracheotomy may be necessary. Overall 21% of patients will require tracheotomy with an associated poor prognosis [5].

## Adjuvant Therapy

Adjuvant therapy is defined as additional treatment offered following a surgical procedure in order to improve the outcome of patients at risk for relapse. In RRP 20% of patients will require adjuvant therapy of some kind [29]. Before discussing specific therapies it is crucial to define when adjuvant therapy should be considered. Adjuvant therapy in RRP may be implemented in the following settings:

1. Four or more surgeries per year.

2. Distal or metastatic disease.

3. Rapid growth resulting in airway compromise.

## CIDOFIVIR

Cidofivir is an antiviral medication that functions as a nucleoside analog of deoxycytidine monophosphate. In its active form it is incorporated into DNA resulting in toxicity of herpes family viruses. Currently, its use is limited by the FDA to the intravenous treatment of cytomegalovirus (CMV) retinitis in HIV positive patients. As a result, any use of cidofivir in RRP represents off-label usage. Typically, therapy involves intralesional injection at the time of surgical therapy. Hopes for the effectiveness of this therapy were spurred by a 10-year systematic review performed by Chadha and colleagues. They demonstrated 57% complete disease resolution and 35% partial resolution [30]. In contrast the only placebo controlled trial to date, performed by McMurray *et al.*, found no difference in Derkay-Coltrera score or subjective symptom score between groups [31]. Both of these studies have flaws. The studies included by Chadha and colleagues in their review lacked randomization and standardization of technique while McMurray's research is limited by small sample size and low dose. These opposing studies demonstrate the need for improvements in this particular field of research. In order to accurately study the effectiveness of cidofivir, randomization and a placebo arm must be included to account for the improvement achieved by surgery alone. In addition dose, interval of therapy and length of trial therapy must all be standardized.

Regardless of effectiveness the potential side effects of cidofivir must be acknowledged and discussed. The classic side effect of cidofivir is nephrotoxicty. It has been proposed that the intralesional use of cidofivir should result in less systemic exposure than in the intravenous treatment of CMV retinitis. Intralesional, cidofivir does appear to have some degree of systemic absorption with 1 of 35 patients in one study approaching systemic nephrotoxic levels [32]. Animal studies involving rats have also shown an increased risk of mammary adenocarcinomas [33]. This finding however, has not been seen in humans or higher level primates [34]. An additional concern centers on the risk for dysplasia. Intralesional therapy is associated with a 2.7% rate of dysplasia [33]. While this is at first glance concerning it fails to differ statistically form the 2.3% spontaneous dysplasia rate in RRP. Before counseling a patient about cidofivir therapy the patient must meet all requirements for adjuvant therapy and be appropriately counseled about possible side effects.

## INTERFERON

Interferon was initially the most common adjuvant therapy in RRP. Interferons are proteins that activate immune response to pathogens and tumor cells. They continue to be used today in the setting of metastatic melanoma. These agents have demonstrated some success with a multicenter non-randomized prospective trial showing 63% of RRP patients with remission at long term followup [35].

However, the effectiveness of this agent is essentially mitigated by its notorious side effects. Common side effects include fever, flu-like symptoms nausea and vomiting. Less common but more severe side effects include growth retardation, liver toxicity, central nervous system side effects and thrombocytopenia. This profile in combination with general poor tolerance of therapy has resulted in infrequent use of interferon in RRP.

## OTHER THERAPIES

As in any difficult to treat disease entity, new and novel therapies are constantly being put forth for the treatment of RRP. The cyclooxygenase-2 (COX-2) inhibitor Celebrex, and GERD therapy have been proposed as medical adjuncts.

Celebrex is thought to target the signaling pathway of HPV infected cells. Favorable anecdotal results have led to an ongoing multi-institutional trial with results pending. Gastroesophageal reflux has long been proposed as a confounding factor in RRP with resultant inflammatory changes. Control of reflux in small case series and retrospective reviews have shown improved response to surgical therapy, and decreased risk of laryngeal web in high risk patients [36-37]. Further randomized controlled trials are necessary to elucidate the real effect of GERD on RRP.

## VACCINATION

### Therapeutic Vaccine

The role of vaccination in the treatment of RRP entails a two-pronged approach. The HspE7 vaccine represents a direct, therapeutic, approach targeting HPV viral proteins E6 and E7. Animal studies have demonstrated that this vaccine is effective in inciting specific humoral immunity, cell mediated immune response and regression of epithelial cell-derived tumor.

Clinical trials have been promising in the treatment of genital warts with phase II trials demonstrating increased surgical interval and decreased need for surgical interventions [38]. The vaccine has also been shown to be well tolerated and easily administered in an outpatient setting. In addition, while HspE7 is produced by cross-linking proteins to the E7 portion of HPV16, it has been demonstrated to be effective on non-HPV16 strains. This cross-reactivity is promising for future therapeutic use, but further research is needed prior to broad implementation.

## Preventative Vaccine

While therapeutic vaccines seem promising a majority of public and academic interest has focused on preventative vaccination. The quadrivalent HPV vaccine (Gardisel TM, Merck and Co, Inc) targets HPV serotype 6, 11, 16 and 18. The potential benefits of such a vaccine are undeniable given that HPV 16 and 18 account for 70% of cervical cancers and HPV 6 and 11 lead to 95% of genital warts [39-40]. The quadrivalent vaccine has been shown to effectively prevent cervical cancer, adenocarcinoma *in situ* and cervical intraepithelial neoplasia as well as vulvar/vaginal intraepithelial neoplasia and HPV genital warts [41]. In the largest randomized double blinded placebo controlled trial to date the Future II study enrolled 12,167 women ages 15-26. Each participant received 3 doses of vaccine or placebo and was followed for 3 years. The vaccine was shown to have 98% efficacy for the prevention of high-grade cervical lesions [42]. There also appeared to be an imperative for early treatment with the vaccination less effective if the patient had intraepithelial lesions prior to enrollment. Based on this research it has been recommended that girls age 11 to 12 and women 13 to 26 be vaccinated. Girls as young as nine may also be vaccinated when deemed appropriate by a physician. The implementation of these recommendations has not thus far been immediate or universal. Based upon data supporting reduced risk for developing genital warts, the FDA has also approved the quadrivalent vaccine for permissive use in boys. It is anticipated that this may also reduce the incidence of penile and anal cancers as well as some oropharyngeal squamous cell carcinomas. While the controversy over universal vaccination has often been portrayed with a focus on moral concerns the real barriers to action involve logistics and cost. Estimates place that the cost of vaccinating all 11 year old females at 850 million dollars per year [43]. While this number seems daunting the reduction in surgical intervention and eventually surveillance clearly appears to be cost effective with every 13 cents spent on prevention resulting in a dollar's saving in treatment and surveillance costs. The effectiveness of the vaccine may be enhanced by the development and use of a 9 valent HPV vaccine currently in clinical trials as well as the achievement of herd immunity. It is estimated that by immunizing 80% of girls, broader herd immunity may be established. Unfortunately, currently only about 27% of girls in the US are being fully vaccinated [44]. While not the driving force for universal vaccination, RRP would no doubt benefit from a reduction or near eradication of HPV 6 and 11. The rarity of RRP will make the effects of vaccination difficult to quantify necessitating many years of dedicated research.

## CONCLUSION

Recurrent respiratory papilloma is a disease that is costly both in individual and societal terms. Children with RRP in academic medical centers may require nearly 20 procedures over the course of their lifetime [11]. This disorder subsequently imposes a direct economic burden of 150 million dollars per year upon society [6]. The pediatrician plays an essential role in both the diagnosis and management of children with RRP. Only through thorough knowledge and astute observation can delay in diagnosis be avoided, appropriate referral initiated, and suffering of this disease alleviated.

## ACKNOWLEDGEMENT

Declared none.

## CONFLICT OF INTEREST

The authors confirm that this chapter content has no conflict of interest.

## REFERENCES

[1]　Silverman EM. Incidence of chronic hoarseness among school-age children. J Speech Hear Disord 1975; 40:211.
[2]　Duff MC, Proctor A, Yairi E. Prevalence of voice disorders in African American and European American preschoolers. J Voice 2004; 18:348.
[3]　Carding PN, Roulstone S, Northstone K, ALSPAC Study Team. The prevalence of childhood dysphonia: a cross-sectional study. J Voice 2006; 20:623.
[4]　Morgan AH, Zitsch RP. Recurrent respiratory papillomatosis in children: a retrospective study of management and complications. *Ear Nose Throat.J* 1986;65:19–28.
[5]　Schraff S, Derkay CS. Burke B, Lawson L (2004) American Society of Pediatric Otolaryngology members' experience with recurrent respiratory papiilomatosis and the use of adjuvant therapy. Arch Otolaryngol Head Neck Surg 130:1039-42.

[6]     [Derkay CS. Task force on recurrent respiratory papillomas. *Arch Otolaryngol Head Neck Surg.* 1995;121:1386–1391.

[7]     [7] Silverman EM. Incidence of chronic hoarseness among school-age children. J Speech Hear Disord 1975; 40:211.

[8]     Buchinsky FJ, Donfack J, Derkay CS, Choi SS, Conley SF, Myer CM III *et al.* (2008) Age of child, more than HPV type, is associated with clinical course in recurrent respiratory papillomatosis. PLoS ONE 28: e2263.

[9]     Mounts P, Shah KV, Kashima H. Viral etiology of juvenile and adult onset squamous papilloma of the larynx. *Proc Natl Acad Sci U S A.* 1982;79:5425–5429.

[10]    Silverberg MJ, Thorsen P, Lindeberg H, Ahdieh-Grant L, Shah KV. Clinical course of RRP in Danish children. *Arch OTO-HNS.* 2004;130:711-7116

[11]    Armstrong LR, Derkay CS, Reeves WC. Initial results from the National Registry for juvenile-onset recurrent respiratory papillomatosis. *Arch Otolaryngol Head Neck Surg.* 1999;125:743–748.

[12]    Cohn AM, Kos JT, Taber LH, Adam E. (1981) Recurring laryngeal papilloma. Am J Otolaryngol. 2:129–32.

[13]    [13] Wiatrak BJ, Wialrak DW. Broker TR. Lewis L. (2004) Recurrent respiratory papillomatosis: a longitudinal study comparing severity associated with human papilloma viral types 6 and 11 and other risk factors in a large pediatric population. Laryngoscope 114:1-23.

[14]    Bennett RS, Powell KR (1987) Human papillomavirus: association between laryngeal papillomas and genital warts. Pediatr Infect Dis J 6:229–32.

[15]    Armstrong LR, Preston EJ, Reichert M, Phillips DL, Nisenbaum R, Todd NW, Jacobs IN, Inglis AF, Manning SC, Reeves WC. Incidence and prevalence of recurrent respiratory papillomatosis among children in Atlanta and Seattle. *Clin Infect Dis.* 2000 Jul;31(1):107-109. Epub 2000 Jul 11.

[16]    Campisi P. The Epidemiology of Juvenile Onset Recurrent Respiratory Papillomatosis Derived From a Population Level National Database. *Laryngoscope.* 2010 (in press).

[17]    Marsico M, Mehta V, Wentworth C, Chastek B, Derkay CS. Estimating the disease burden of juvenile onset RRP in the US using large administrative databases – preliminary pilot results. Presented May 2009 at the International Papillomavirus Conference. http://www.hpv2009.org. abstract P-03.58.

[18]    Leung R, Hawkes M, Campisi. Severity of juvenile onset recurrent respiratory papillomatosis is not associated with socioeconomic status in a setting of universal health care. *Intl J Ped Otorhinol.* 2007; 71:965-972.

[19]    Lindman J, Lewis L, Accortt, Wiatrak, BJ. Use of the pediatric quality of life inventory to assess the health related qualiy of life in children with recurrent respiratory papillomatosis. *Ann Otol Rhino Laryngol.* 2005; 114: 499-503.

[20]    Kashima HK. Shah F. Lyics A. *et al.* (1992) A comparison of risk factors in juvenile-onset and adult-onset recurrent respiratory papiilomatosis. Laryngoscope 102:9-13.

[21]    Lindeberg H, Elbrond O. Laryngeal papillomas: the epidemiology in a Danish subpopulation 1965–1984. *Clin Otolaryngol.* 1991;15:125–131.

[22]    Rimell FL, Shoemaker DL, Pou AM, *et al.* Pediatric respiratory papillomatosis: prognostic role of viral subtyping and cofactors. *Laryngoscope.* 1997;107:915–918.

[23]    Tenti P, Zappatore R, Migliora P, Spinillo A, Belloni C, Carnevali L. Perinatal transmission of human papillomavirus from gravidas with latest infections. *Obstet Gynecol.* 1999;93:475-479.

[24]    Derkay CS, Malis DJ, Zalzal G, Wiatrak BJ, Kashima HK, Coltera MD (1998) A staging system for assessing severity of disease and response to therapy in recurrent respiratory papillomatosis. Laryngoscope 108:935-7

[25]  Hester RP, Derkay CS, Burke BL, Lawson ML (2003) Reliability of a staging assessment system for recurrent respiratory papillomatosis. Int J Pediatr Otorhinolaryngol. 67:505-9

[26]  Zeitels SM. Sataloff RT (1999) Phonomicrosurgical resection of glottal papillomatosis. J Voice 13:123-7.

[27]  Pasquale K, Wiatrak B, Woolley A, Lewis L (2003) Microdebrider *versus* CO2 laser removal of recurrent respiratory papillomas: a prospective analysis. Laryngoscope. 113(1):139-43.

[28]  Holler T, Allegro J, Chadha NK, Hawkes M, Harrison RV, Forte V, Campisi P (2009) Voice outcomes following repeated surgical resection of laryngeal papillomata in children. Otolaryngol Head Neck Surg. 141(4):522-6.

[29]  Sajan A, Kerschner J, Merati A. Prevalence of dysplasia in juvenile onset recurrent respiratory papillomatosis. *Arch Otolaryngol Head Neck Surg.* 2010; 136: 7-11.

[30]  Chadha NK, James AL. Antiviral agents for the treatment of recurrent respiratory papillomatosis: a systematic review of the English-language literature. *Cochrane Review.* 2007; 136(6):863-869.

[31]  McMurray JS, Conner N, Ford C. Cidofovir efficacy in RRP: a prospective blinded placebo-controlled study. *Annals Otol Rhinol Laryngol.* 2008;117:477-483.

[32]  Naiman A, Roger G, Marie-Claude *et al.* Cidofovir plasma assays after local injection in respiratory papillomatosis. *Laryngoscope.* 2004; 114:1151-1156.

[33]  http://www.fda.gov/cder/foi/adcomm/96/avdac_joint_031496_summmin_ac.pdf

[34]  Lacy S, Hitchcock M, Lee W, Tellier P, Cundy K. Effect of oral probenecid coadministration on the chronic toxicity and pharmacokinetics of intravenous cidofovir in cynomolgus monkeys. *Toxicol Sci.* 1889; 44(2):97-106.

[35]  Gerein V, Rastirguev E, Gerein J, *et al.* (2005) Use of interferon-alpha in recurrent respiratory papillomatosis: 20 year follow-up. Ann Otol Rhinol Laryngol 114:463-71

[36]  Derkay C, Wiatrak B. Recurrent respiratory papillomatosis: a review. *Laryngoscope.* 2008;118(7):1236-1247.

[37]  McKenna M, Brodsky L. Extraesophageal acid reflux and recurrent respiratory papilloma in children. *Int. J. Ped. Otorhinolaryngol.* 2005; 69:597-605.

[38]  Rosen C, Bryson P. Indole-3-carbinol for recurrent respiratory papillomatosis: long-term results. *J Voice.* 2004;18:248-253.

[39]  Duff MC, Proctor A, Yairi E. Prevalence of voice disorders in African American and European American preschoolers. J Voice 2004; 18:348.

[40]  Carding PN, Roulstone S, Northstone K, ALSPAC Study Team. The prevalence of childhood dysphonia: a cross-sectional study. J Voice 2006; 20:623.

[41]  Zeitels, SM, Lopez-Guerra G, Burns JA *et al.* Microlaryngoscopic and Office-Based Injection of Bevacizumab (Avastin) to Enhance 532-nm Pulsed KTP Laser Treatment of Glottal Papillomatosis. *Ann Otol Rhinol Laryngol.* 2009;118;1-24.

[42]  FUTURE II Study Group (2007) Quadrivalent vaccine against HPV to prevent high-grade cervical lesions. N Engl J Med 356:1915-27

[43]  Freed GL. Derkay CS. Prevention of RRP: the role of HPV vaccination. *Intl J Ped Otorhinol.* 2007;70;1799-1803.

[44]  Markowitz L, HPV vaccines—prophylactic, not therapeutic. *JAMA.* 2007;298;805-806.

*Send Orders of Reprints at reprints@benthamscience.net*

*Otolaryngology for the Pediatrician, 2013, 178-197*

# CHAPTER 12

# Approach and Management of Congenital Vascular Anomalies

## Nitin J. Patel[1] and Nancy M. Bauman[2,*]

*[1]Division of Otolaryngology, George Washington University, 111 Michigan Avenue, 20010 NW, Washington, D.C., USA and [2]Children's National Medical Center, George Washington University, 111 Michigan Avenue, 20010 NW, Washington, D.C., USA*

**Abstract:** Congenital vascular anomalies are a heterogeneous group of lesions that may occur as isolated findings or as part of a constellation of symptoms or syndrome. These anomalies are divided into vascular tumors or vascular malformations depending on the growth rate of their constituent cells. Infantile hemangiomas are vascular tumors and are the most common of the vascular anomalies followed by capillary malformations, lymphatic malformations, venous malformations and arteriovenous malformations. Proper diagnosis is critical for appropriate management of these enigmatic lesions. Diagnosis is usually readily secured by history and physical findings although imaging studies are sometimes necessary. Management varies considerably depending on the nature of the lesion, its propensity for growth and its physical impact. Observation is appropriate for some vascular anomalies, while others require pharmacologic treatment, sclerotherapy, embolization, laser treatment or surgical excision. Nearly all patients with vascular anomalies should be seen by a physician or team of physicians who specializes in the care of these unique disorders.

**Keywords:** Vascular anomaly, vascular tumor, infantile hemangioma, congenital hemangioma, PHACES, Kaposiform hemangioendothelioma, Kassabach Merritt phenomenon, capillary malformation, tufted angioma, lymphatic malformation, venous malformation, arteriovenous malformation.

## CLASSIFICATION OF VASCULAR ANOMALIES

Congenital vascular anomalies comprise a heterogeneous group of vascular lesions. The terminology used to describe these lesions was notoriously haphazard until 1982 when Glowacki and Mulliken proposed a classification scheme

***Address correspondence to Nancy M. Bauman:** Children's National Medical Center, George Washington University, 111 Michigan Avenue, 2000 NW, Washington, D.C., USA; Tel: 202 476-3712; Fax: 202 476-5038; E-mail: nbauman@cnmc.org

distinguishing vascular tumors from vascular malformations based primarily on the activity of the endothelial cell, a universal constituent of vascular lesions [1]. The endothelial cells of vascular tumors, such as the relatively common infantile hemangioma, grow more rapidly than their host body. The endothelial cells of vascular malformations, such as lymphatic malformations, generally grow at a similar rate of their host body although the lesions can enlarge rapidly in the face of infection or hormonal changes. Despite the congenital nature of these lesions, vascular malformations may not always be apparent until adolescence, or even adulthood.

The distinguishing growth and clinical features of the more common vascular anomalies are described in this chapter, including infantile hemangiomas, Kaposiform hemangioendotheliomas, tufted angiomas and lymphatic, capillary, venous and arteriovenous malformations. While the diagnosis of most vascular anomalies can be obtained *via* a thorough history and clinical examination, the diagnosis of rare lesions can be difficult and a delay in diagnosis can have devastating sequelae. Patients with complex vascular anomalies should undergo an initial evaluation in a multidisciplinary vascular anomalies clinic available at most tertiary care institutions to confirm the diagnosis, discuss management and, most importantly, determine if diagnostic studies are indicated to exclude other concomitant anomalies. A recent review of over 5000 patients evaluated in a well established vascular anomaly center revealed that only 53% of congenital vascular lesions were correctly diagnosed prior to referral [2].

## VASCULAR TUMORS

### Infantile Hemangiomas

Infantile hemangiomas (IH) are not only the most common of the vascular anomalies but also the most common tumor of infancy with an estimated incidence of 10% [3]. IH arise in females far more commonly than males with a ratio of 4:1 and are more common in caucasian infants and in infants that are premature, of low birth weight, of multiple gestation or born to mothers of advanced age [4].

Interestingly, IH are usually not apparent at birth, or are heralded by a seemingly innocuous premonitory vascular blush. They have a unique growth pattern characterized by 4 stages beginning with a proliferative phase that usually begins during the first several weeks of life. The proliferative stage is divided into a rapidly proliferative phase, peaking around 4 months of age and a slower proliferative phase that usually continues until 12 months of age, and sometimes longer for particularly large lesions (Fig. **1**) [5]. IH remain relatively unchanged during the plateau stage before they begin to regress during the involuting stage. When involution appears stable and unchanged, the lesion is in the final phase, or the involuted phase.

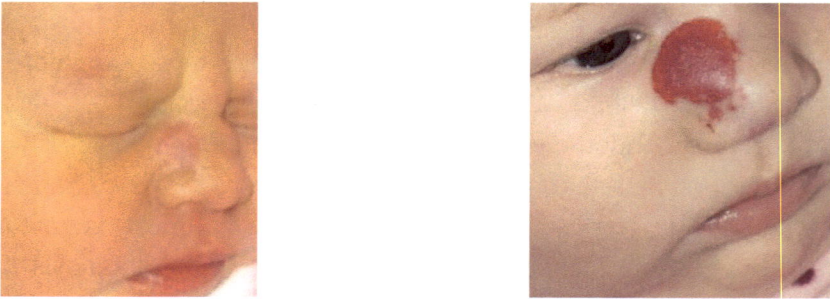

**Figure 1:** Vascular blush of early IH of right nasal bridge at 2 weeks of age (left). Same IH in rapidly proliferative phase at 2 months of age (right).

It is generally believed from much earlier reports that 50% of lesions are fully involuted by age 5, 70% by age 7, and 90% by age 9 [6]. This data is quite easy to relay to parents and is widely quoted despite the absence of subsequent supportive studies. What is generally not relayed to parents is that fully involuted lesions often appear as fibrofatty tissue that can be particularly disfiguring depending on the size and location of the original IH (Fig. **2**).

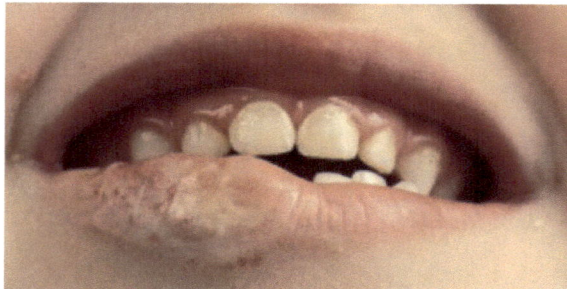

**Figure 2:** Cosmetically deforming fibrofatty tissue of untreated fully involuted lip IH. Early pharmacologic treatment of this "asymptomatic" IH would likely have improved cosmetic outcome.

Over 2/3 of IH arise in the head and neck, 23% on the trunk, 18% on the extremities and 6% in the perineum [7]. In 30% of cases, multiple lesions are present. IH are further subdivided into focal, segmental or indeterminate lesions depending on their extent of involvement [6]. Focal lesions are discrete while segmental lesions involve an entire segment of development such as the maxillary, mandibular, frontotemporal or frontonasal regions [8]. Most hemangiomas are superficial or mixed lesions that affect the epidermis of the skin. Deep hemangiomas often require imaging studies to visualize their full extent.

IH are differentiated from the far less common "congenital hemangiomas" that may have a similar clinical appearance but do not show the characteristic growth patterns of IH. Congenital hemangiomas are fully apparent at birth and do not proliferate. The two types of congenital hemangiomas have markedly varied patterns of involution with "RICH" (rapidly involuting congenital hemangiomas) regressing by 12-14 months of age and "NICH" (non-involuting congenital hemangiomas) failing to regress [9,10]. Correct diagnosis is critical to management and sometimes requires biopsy with immunohistochemistry staining for glucose transport protein receptor (glut-1) that is widely present in IH but lacking in congenital hemangiomas [11]. The recognition of congenital hemangiomas significantly improved the ability to classify the growth patterns of all hemangiomas.

The etiology of IH is unknown. Most investigators believe that IH arise from defects in angiogenesis, [12,13] others believe that they arise from clonal expansions of endothelial cells with mutated growth regulatory genes, [14] while still others hypothesize that they arise from embolized fetal placental endothelial cells since they share transcriptomes with placental tissue [15,16,17].

IH may occur as isolated phenomenon or as part of a constellation of anomalies. The most common constellation is designated by the acronym PHACES characterized by Posterior fossa malformations, Hemangiomas, Arterial anomalies, Coarctation of the aorta/Cardiac defects, Eye abnormalities, and Sternal or abdominal clefting [18]. A significant number of infants with large (>5 cm) segmental hemangiomas of the face, scalp and neck are at risk of having PHACES and may manifest only one of the associated anomalies. The female:

male ratio of PHACES is 9:1. Infants at risk of PHACES should undergo a thorough history and physical examination, ophthalmic evaluation, echocardiogram and MRI of the head and neck. The ipsilateral internal carotid artery is the most frequently involved intracranial artery and in very rare instances acute ischemic events associated with narrowing have been reported [19,20]. "SACRAL" should be considered in patients with IH of the sacral area who may also have anomalies of the bony sacrum, imperforate anus, renal anomalies abnormal genitalia and leptomeningomyeloceles [21,22].

Cutaneous IH in the "beard distribution" have a high incidence of an associated subglottic hemangioma that may be life-threatening if unrecognized. Consequently, any infant with such a hemangioma who manifests stridor, wheezing, or "raspy" breathing should be referred to an otolaryngologist immediately for an urgent or emergent direct laryngoscopy and bronchoscopy depending on the nature of the symptoms (Fig. **3**).

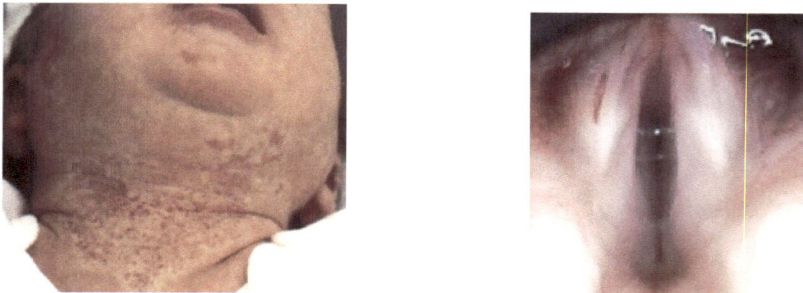

**Figure 3:** Early IH in beard distribution in 3 week old infant (left). Tracheotomy required due to bilateral subglottic hemangioma (right) and failure to respond to pharmacologic therapy. Note markedly narrowed subglottis just inferior to vocal cords.

Patients with liver hemangiomas, particularly when diffuse, are at risk of hypothyroidism due to high levels of type 3 iodothryonine [23,24]. Most intrahepatic hemangiomas are diagnosed on prenatal ultrasound and remain completely asymptomatic generally disappearing within the first year of life [25].

Since involution is the expected outcome of IH, only 10-35% require therapy other than observation [26,27]. IH warranting treatment are more likely to be large lesions, lesions located on the face, ulcerated lesions or lesions that affect normal infant functions including respiration, vision, hearing, eating, micturition, defecation, and limb mobility [6]. Lesions that ulcerate should be treated since ulceration is painful and portends a poor cosmetic outcome. Most of these indications are relatively readily apparent while the need to treat other lesions is less easily recognized. Size alone is not an indication for treatment since even small lesions can cause devastating alterations in normal development and leave an unsightly, emotionally disturbing deformity that requires surgical reconstruction. Examples of this are lesions of the nasal tip that may measure less than a centimeter in diameter but that compress and permanently disfigure the underlying cartilaginous framework causing enduring cosmetic deformity. This recognition further supports the value of an evaluation by a multidisciplinary vascular anomaly team early in infancy when treatment is most efficacious. A delay in treatment may negatively impact an infant's ultimate outcome.

Historically, systemic or intralesional corticosteroids were the most commonly prescribed medications for treating symptomatic IH. Although outcome data is quite limited, the "rule of 1/3's" is generally quoted to parents when discussing the efficacy of corticosteroids. Active shrinkage occurs in approximately 33% of patients, nearly 40% have an 'equivocal' response, where it is difficult to separate the effect of corticosteroids from the natural progression of the disease and the remainder have continued growth [28]. Side effects of corticosteroids include increased appetite, irritability, Cushingnoid features, systemic hypertension, delayed linear growth, immunosuppression, delayed wound healing [29]. and potentially life-threatening adrenal insufficiency if stopped suddenly (Fig. **4**).

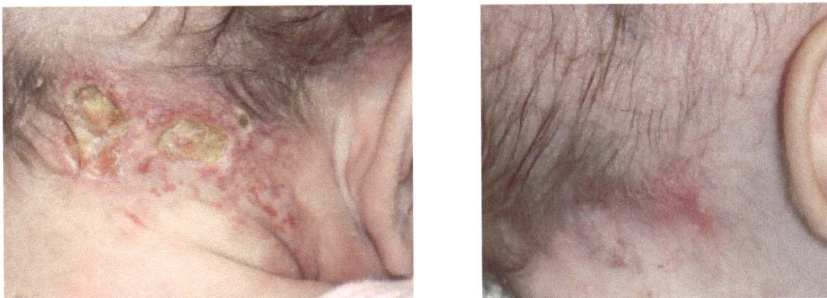

**Figure 4:** Ulcerated, painful IH of right posterior neck and scalp (left). Marked improvement after 3 months of corticosteroid use (right).

The 2008 serendipitous discovery of propranolol's efficacy in treating IH is dramatically challenging the use of corticosteroids [30]. Since the initial report of

11 patients, propranolol is now considered the first line treatment for most IH by most clinicians [31]. Propranolol has an attractive, relatively low side-effect profile and has been used in pediatric cardiology for 40 years, although, as is true for corticosteroids, its use for this indication is off label. Potential side effects include bradycardia, bronchospasm, hypotension, hypersomnolence, gastroesophageal reflux, altered sleep and hypoglycemia that can be severe enough to induce seizure activity [32-34]. The rate of adverse events in this population is estimated at 18% [35] but serious adverse effects are rare and propranolol currently appears better tolerated than corticosteroids and at least equally effective [30]. Although up to 2/3 of infants started on propranolol will experience bradycardia or hypotension during their initiation, the events are typically asymptomatic and resolve without the need for therapy. A prospective clinical trial comparing the efficacy and adverse events of prednisolone *versus* propranolol is underway [34] (ClinicalTrials.gov NCT00967226) and guidelines for initiating and monitoring propranolol from the Multidisciplinary Propranolol Guidelines Conference held December, 2011 in Chicago, IL were recently published [36].

Treatment with propranolol is often required until near complete involution or at least until a year of age to reduce the risk of rebound growth [32,36]. Results of the prospective clinical trial noted above may reveal that propranolol treatment is required for longer than corticosteroids to induce permanent involution. Propranolol appears to be effective even when administered after the proliferative phase of growth [37]. Future studies will confirm whether early reports advocating topical timolol for select IH are reproducible [38-40].

Although interferon alpha is effective in inducing early involution of IH, it is rarely used today due to the risk of inducing spastic diplegia when administered to young infants [41,42].

## Kaposiform Hemangioendothelioma and Tufted Angiomas

Kaposiform hemangioendotheliomas (KHEs) and tufted angiomas (TAs) are non-hemangioma vascular tumors. KHEs and TAs occur anywhere in the head and neck. Interestingly, these vascular tumors can have a significant lymphatic component in addition to blood vascular endothelium [43]. Their pathology is characterized by endothelial cells in nodules which are CD31, CD34 and FL11 positive but negative for GLUT1, HHV-8 d240, and prox 1 – distinguishing these lesions from lymphatic malformations, hemangiomas and Kaposi sarcomas [43-46].

Clinically, KHEs appear as violaceous cutaneous nodules that infiltrate deep tissues locally. Radiographically, KHEs show diffuse infiltrative vascular processes. TAs are more localized and may or may not involve the skin. In addition to clinical and radiographic findings, diagnosis usually requires incisional biopsy with immunohistochemical staining.

In children, the primary morbidity from KHEs and TAs is from mass effect and platelet consumption in the form of Kasabach-Merritt phenomenon [47]. Kasabach-Merritt phenomenon is the occurrence of thrombocytopenia in association with vascular tumors. KHE and TA, not IH, are the vascular tumors most associated with Kasabach-Merritt phenomenon. The mechanism leading to profound thrombocytopenia is unknown and the spectrum of this phenomenon is still being defined.

Treatment for both KHE's and TA's is centered on prevention of complications and tumor control. For localized tumors, curative surgical resection is possible. However, for larger tumors with extensive tumor infiltration across tissue planes and significant risk of morbidity or morality from bleeding or for those that are associated with the development of Kasabach-Merritt, chemotherapy may be necessary. Other treatments have included corticosteroids, radiation, anti-inflammatory agents and anti-angiogenic agents including interferon and sirolimus [48-55]. No standard of care has been established.

## VASCULAR MALFORMATIONS

Congenital vascular malformations may arise from any component of the vascular system, namely from the lymphatics, capillaries, veins, and/or arteries. Vascular malformations are characterized by the nature of their flow. Low flow lesions include anomalies of the lymphatics, capillary, and/or venous systems and components of all three of these systems often coexist within a lesion. High flow lesions have an arterial feeder and lack a normal intervening capillary bed. The more common vascular malformations are discussed here.

## Lymphatic Malformations

Lymphatic malformations (LMs) are benign congenital lesions that arise from aberrant development of the lymphatic system. The lymphatic system first appears as outpouchings of the venous system that coalesce to form connecting channels. LMs arise if these primordial sacs and channels fail to maintain communication with the central venous system and sequester themselves independently [56].

LMs are classified as macrocystic, microcystic or mixed lesions depending on their dominant component. By definition, macrocysts are cysts greater than 2 cc in volume [57]. Macrocystic LMs were once referred to as "cystic hygromas" and microcystic LMs as "lymphangiomas", but these historic, non-descriptive and confusing terms should no longer be used. Generally, macrocystic LMs are far easier to treat than microcystic lesions (Fig. **5**).

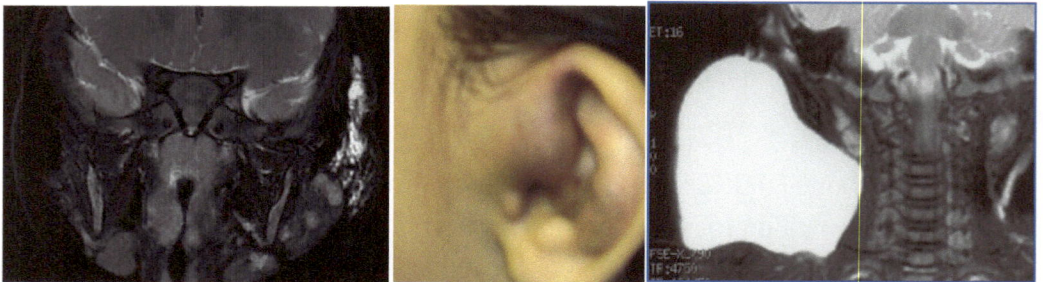

**Figure 5:** T2 weighted coronal MR of left peri-auricular microcystic LM (left and middle). T2 weighted coronal MR of large right cervical macrocystic LM (right). Note multiple septations in microcystic lesion compared to macrocystic lesion. Septations presumably limit the efficacy of sclerotherapy.

Similar to IH, 70% of LMs arise in the head and neck region. Approximately half are present birth and 90% by 2 years of age with the remaining lesions even arising in adult patients [58]. Unlike IH, spontaneous involution is the exception and not the rule, occurring in fewer than 15% of cases and only in macrocystic LMs [59]. More common than involution is a temporary increase in size that may occur after an upper respiratory infection or following intralesional hemorrhage that arises from spontaneous disruption of the aberrantly developed veins within the walls of the LM.

Cervical LMs are staged based on their relationship to the hyoid bone. Stage I lesions are unilateral and infrahyoid, stage II are unilateral and suprahyoid, stage

III are unilateral and both infra- and suprahyoid, stage IV are bilateral and suprahyoid and stage V are bilateral and both infra- and suprahyoid [60]. The higher the stage, the more difficult the LM is to treat.

LMs are usually readily diagnosed based on their clinical appearance. They are soft, non-tender, non-fluctuant masses. Macrocystic LMs transilluminate more readily than microcystic lesions whose septations often prevent light transmission. Macrocystic LMs have well-defined margins but microcystic lesions are poorly circumscribed with extensions that insinuate themselves around adjacent vessels and nerves in a challenging fashion. Imaging studies are sometimes indicated for diagnosis but are more often obtained to determine the deep extent of the lesion. For this latter reason, magnetic resonance or computed tomography is preferred over ultrasound imaging.

LM's can be observed or treated depending on their site, their symptoms, and their prognosis for complete extirpation without significant nerve injury. Treatment is generally recommended when feasible to prevent the risk of spontaneous infection or to treat the cosmetic impairment. Macrocystic LMs are amenable to surgical excision or to clerotherapy, which seems equally efficacious and less invasive. A variety of agents have been utilized as LM sclerosants with the most common being OK432 (picibinal), doxycycline, and ethanol (Fig. **6**) [57, 61, 62-65]. Treating microcystic lesions is far more complex since they require surgical excision and their margins are so poorly defined. Injuries to nerves incorporated within massive microcystic lesions are common as are recurrences since complete extirpation is difficult to achieve [59, 66]. Sadly, control of the lesion rather than eradication is sometimes the more realistic outcome.

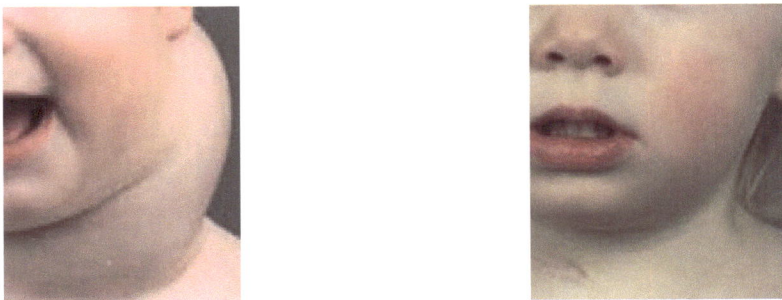

**Figure 6:** Large left cervical macrocystic LM before (left) and after (right) OK432 sclerotherapy.

Immunosuppressive agents such as rapamycin may prove effective as adjuvant therapy. The author's personal experience with sildenfail therapy is limited but results have not been encouraging.

## Capillary Malformations

Capillary malformations (CM) are comprised of malformed capillary vessels and include port wine stains, capillary lymphatic malformations, telangiectasias and cutis marmorata telangiectasia congenita [67]. Port wine stain is the most common vascular malformation affecting an estimated 0.6% of live births [68]. Port wine stains appear during infancy as macular, pink cutaneous stains with well defined border. These low flow lesions gradually darken over the course of a lifetime. The most notable capillary malformation was that on the forehead of Mikhail Gorbachav, former President of the former Soviet Union and 1990 Nobel Peace Prize recipient.

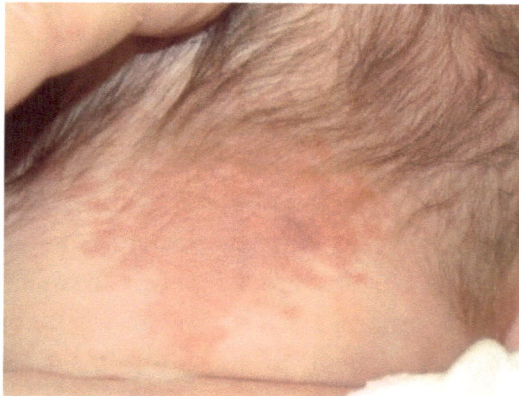

**Figure 7:** Stork bite in characteristic posterior neck location.

Port wine stains must be differentiated from other vascular appearing macular stains of infancy. These other lesions are known by a variety of names including stork bite, salmon patch, angel's kiss or naevus flammeus neonatoruum. Unlike port wine stains, these lesions usually fade within the first year of life and are often located in characteristic locations including the posterior neck, glabella and eyelids (Fig. **7**).

CM are usually isolated lesions, but when located in the V1 or the V1/V2 distribution may be a component of Sturge Weber syndrome characterized by ipsilateral anomalies of the choroid plexus and leptomeninges, glaucoma and seizures [69]. Because of this association, infants with CM involving V1 distribution should undergo MR imaging of the brain. CMs may also occur in association with high flow lesions as noted in Parkes Weber syndrome or with soft tissue hypertrophy as seen in Klippel Trenaunay Weber syndrome. Mutation of the RASA1 gene on chromosome 5 may cause CMs that occur in association with AVMs or arteriovenous fistulae [70]. Port wine stains are best treated with serial laser therapy.

Klippel-Trenaunay-Weber syndrome is characterized by the clinical triad of capillary malformations, soft tissue and bony hypertrophy of the lower extremities and lymphatic or venous malformations with venous varicosities, although not all components have to be present for diagnosis (Fig. **8**) [71]. Most cases are managed conservatively with the need for lifelong compressive stockings. Sclerotherapy and surgical intervention are sometimes indicated.

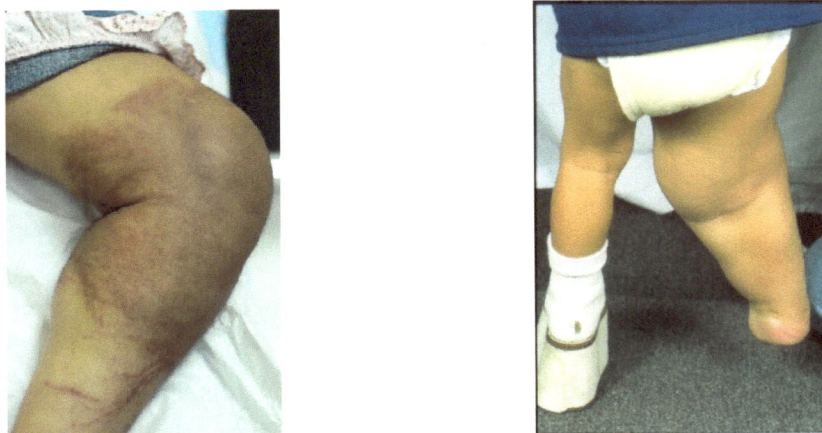

**Figure 8:** Capillary malformations of lower extremities (left) and Klippel-Trenaunay-Weber syndrome (right) demonstrating soft tissue hypertrophy and leg discrepancy.

## Venous Malformations

Venous malformations may appear as isolated spongy masses, or more commonly in combination with anomalies of other aspects of the vascular system. They may be confined to the skin, mucosa, muscles, pelvis, chest, abdominal cavity, visceral organs or brain. Venous malformations are four times more common than arteriovenous malformations and in 90% of cases are present at birth, affecting an estimated 0.2% of live births. They affect males and females equally, and generally show normal endothelial cell growth commensurate with the child. Marked increases in growth can occur during certain periods that appear to have hormonal influence including puberty, pregnancy, or even initiation of birth control pills.

Isolated venous malformations have distinctive clinical findings. They lend a bluish hue to the overlying skin or mucosa, are spongy to palpation and characteristically engorge when placed in the dependent position (Fig. **9**). Unlike high flow lesions, they are easily compressible, refill slowly upon release and lack a bruit or thrill. Over the course of time, venous malformations tend to develop phleboliths that are firm to palpation and often painful.

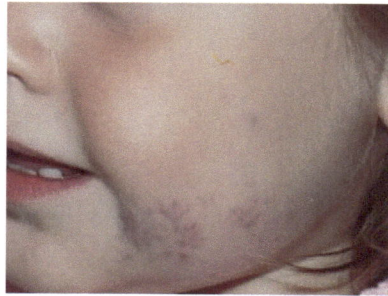

**Figure 9:** Venous malformation of left cheek and chin.

Isolated venous malformations are usually treated by direct percutaneous sclerotherapy with sodium tetradecyl sulfate or ethanol which immediately denatures the proteins and destroys endothelial cells [72]. It is generally completed with general anesthesia as it is a painful procedure. Depending on the size of the lesions staged treatment is sometimes necessary due to the dose-related risk of potentially life-threatening acute pulmonary hypertension [73]. Complications of ethanol therapy include tissue necrosis with sloughing of the overlying skin or mucosa, deep venous thrombosis, and injury to adjacent sensory or motor nerves [72].

## Arteriovenous Malformations

Arteriovenous Malformations (AVMs) are high-flow, abnormal communications between arteries and veins that bypass the capillary bed. These lesions are rare anomalies of vascular development and are thought to arise from the failure of arteriovenous channels to undergo apoptosis or regress into the embroyonic precursors to normal vasculature. This 'nidus' of aberrant arterial-venous shunts subsequently canalizes and grows from recruitment and collateralization of nearby vessels.

The exact incidence of AVMs is unknown, although it has been estimated at approximately 5% of vascular anomalies. So far, predilection of AVMs for race or sex has not been demonstrated. Local and diffuse AVMs have been described, with the latter being more common. Focal AVMs have discrete borders with a single arterial feeder and well-defined nidus. Diffuse AVMs span tissue boundaries. These vascular lesions have a predilection for the face, especially the cheek, auricle and oral cavity, and limbs and involve both superficial and deep structures including skin, fat, muscle and even bone [74].

The distinguishing feature of AVMs from other vascular malformations is the presence of high blood flow. These high flow lesions are usually warm to the tough, are pulsatile and often, although not always, have a thrill or bruit present. They are firmer than venous malformations and when compressed fill rapidly. Furthermore, dependent position or valsalva efforts will not result in changes in size as seen with venous malformations. In children, AVMs are most often dormant and progression typically occurs in adolescence or adulthood [75]. The concept of quiescence and subsequent expansion or progression has led to a staging system for AVM, which also identifies the potential long-term sequelae of these vascular lesions. They are staged by the following 4 stages, Stage I Quiescence, a pink or bluish stain; Stage II, Expansion where the lesion is starting to enlarge and pulsations or thrill is present; Stage III Destructive phase where patients develop ulceration, persistent pain, bleeding and destruction of normal tissue and finally Stage 4 Decompensation where cardiac enlargement is present.

Radiological imaging also aids in the diagnosis of AVMs and serves to delineate the extent of involvement with normal tissue. Arteriogram is the gold standard for diagnosing arteriovenous malformations but magnetic resonance angiography is less invasive and an excellent study to differentiate congenital vascular anomalies. Hypolucent arterial flow voids in a diffuse vascular anomaly are highly suggestive of an AVM. Arteriography can be useful in identifying feeding vessels of the central nidus and allows for subsequent selective embolization if desired as a treatment option. Lastly, computed tomography arteriograms (CTAs) have emerged as a useful diagnostic tool for AVMs. This technique can define the morphology, nidus and supportive vasculature of AVMs more specifically than other modalities.

Arteriovenous malformations in children are rare but devastating if left untreated. No reports of spontaneous resolution of AVMs have been described. Ultimately, the relentless growth of these vascular lesions requires early intervention with surgical or embolic management. High flow lesions are extremely difficult to manage since they are only cured if the nidus is effectively removed or destroyed completely. While embolization appears effective in reducing the size of AVMs, lifetime long term data to determine the success of therapy is limited. Complete surgical resection with preoperative embolization appears to lead to better control and management of AVMs and offers the best outcomes for these potentially devastating lesions [75].

## ACKNOWLEDGEMENT

Authors thank Margie Brown for her administrative assistance in the preparation of this Chapter.

## CONFLICT OF INTEREST

None declared.

## DISCLOSURE

The corresponding author receives funding from the NIH for study of hemangiomas (ClinicalTrials.gov NCT00967226).

## REFERENCES

[1]   Mulliken JB, Glowacki J. Hemangiomas and vascular malformations in infants and children: a classification based on endothelial characteristics. *Plast Reconstr Surg.* Mar 1982;69(3):412-422.
[2]   Greene AK, Liu AS, Mulliken JB, Chalache K, Fishman SJ. Vascular anomalies in 5,621 patients: guidelines for referral. *J Pediatr Surg.* Sep;46(9):1784-1789.

[3]     Jacobs AH, Walton RG. The incidence of birthmarks in the neonate. *Pediatrics. August* 1976;58(2):218-222.

[4]     Hemangioma Investigator G, Haggstrom AN, Drolet BA, *et al.* Prospective study of infantile hemangiomas: demographic, prenatal, and perinatal characteristics. *Journal of Pediatrics. March* 2007;150(3):291-294.

[5]     Chang LC, Haggstrom AN, Drolet BA, *et al.* Growth characteristics of infantile hemangiomas: implications for management. *Pediatrics.* Aug 2008;122(2):360-367.

[6]     Jacobs AH. Strawberry hemangiomas; the natural history of the untreated lesion. *Calif Med.* Jan 1957;86(1):8-10.

[7]     Haggstrom AN, Drolet BA, Baselga E, *et al.* Prospective study of infantile hemangiomas: clinical characteristics predicting complications and treatment. *Pediatrics.* Sep 2006;118(3):882-887.

[8]     Haggstrom AN, Lammer EJ, Schneider RA, Marcucio R, Frieden IJ. Patterns of infantile hemangiomas: new clues to hemangioma pathogenesis and embryonic facial development. *Pediatrics.* Mar 2006;117(3):698-703.

[9]     Boon LM, Enjolras O, Mulliken JB. Congenital hemangioma: evidence of accelerated involution. *J Pediatr.* Mar 1996;128(3):329-335.

[10]    Enjolras O, Mulliken JB, Boon LM, Wassef M, Kozakewich HP, Burrows PE. Noninvoluting congenital hemangioma: a rare cutaneous vascular anomaly. *Plast Reconstr Surg.* Jun 2001;107(7):1647-1654.

[11]    North PE, Waner M, Mizeracki A, Mihm MC, Jr. GLUT1: a newly discovered immunohistochemical marker for juvenile hemangiomas. *Hum Pathol.* Jan 2000;31(1):11-22.

[12]    Dadras SS, North PE, Bertoncini J, Mihm MC, Detmar M. Infantile hemangiomas are arrested in an early developmental vascular differentiation state. *Mod Pathol.* Sep 2004;17(9):1068-1079.

[13]    Nguyen VA, Kutzner H, Furhapter C, Tzankov A, Sepp N. Infantile hemangioma is a proliferation of LYVE-1-negative blood endothelial cells without lymphatic competence. *Mod Pathol.* Feb 2006;19(2):291-298.

[14]    Boye E, Yu Y, Paranya G, Mulliken JB, Olsen BR, Bischoff J. Clonality and altered behavior of endothelial cells from hemangiomas. *J Clin Invest.* Mar 2001;107(6):745-752.

[15]    Barnes CM, Huang S, Kaipainen A, *et al.* Evidence by molecular profiling for a placental origin of infantile hemangioma. *Proc Natl Acad Sci U S A.* Dec 27 2005;102(52):19097-19102.

[16]    North PE, Waner M, Mizeracki A, *et al.* A unique microvascular phenotype shared by juvenile hemangiomas and human placenta. *Arch Dermatol.* May 2001;137(5):559-570.

[17]    Burton BK, Schulz CJ, Angle B, Burd LI. An increased incidence of haemangiomas in infants born following chorionic villus sampling (CVS). *Prenat Diagn.* Mar 1995;15(3):209-214.

[18]    Frieden IJ, Reese V, Cohen D. PHACE syndrome. The association of posterior fossa brain malformations, hemangiomas, arterial anomalies, coarctation of the aorta and cardiac defects, and eye abnormalities. *Arch Dermatol.* Mar 1996;132(3):307-311.

[19]    Burrows PE, Robertson RL, Mulliken JB, *et al.* Cerebral vasculopathy and neurologic sequelae in infants with cervicofacial hemangioma: report of eight patients. *Radiology.* Jun 1998;207(3):601-607.

[20]    Metry DW, Dowd CF, Barkovich AJ, Frieden IJ. The many faces of PHACE syndrome. *J Pediatr.* Jul 2001;139(1):117-123.

[21]    Stockman A, Boralevi F, Taieb A, Leaute-Labreze C. SACRAL syndrome: spinal dysraphism, anogenital, cutaneous, renal and urologic anomalies, associated with an angioma of lumbosacral localization. *Dermatology.* 2007;214(1):40-45.

[22]    Goldberg NS, Hebert AA, Esterly NB. Sacral hemangiomas and multiple congenital abnormalities. *Arch Dermatol.* Jun 1986;122(6):684-687.

[23]    Huang SA, Tu HM, Harney JW, *et al.* Severe hypothyroidism caused by type 3 iodothyronine deiodinase in infantile hemangiomas. *N Engl J Med.* Jul 20 2000;343(3):185-189.

[24]    Christison-Lagay ER, Burrows PE, Alomari A, *et al.* Hepatic hemangiomas: subtype classification and development of a clinical practice algorithm and registry. *J Pediatr Surg.* Jan 2007;42(1):62-67; discussion 67-68.

[25]    Dickie B, Dasgupta R, Nair R, *et al.* Spectrum of hepatic hemangiomas: management and outcome. *J Pediatr Surg.* Jan 2009;44(1):125-133.

[26]    Drolet BA, Esterly NB, Frieden IJ. Hemangiomas in children. *N Engl J Med.* Jul 15 1999;341(3):173-181.

[27]    Enjolras O, Gelbert F. Superficial hemangiomas: associations and management. *Pediatr Dermatol.* May-Jun 1997;14(3):173-179.

[28]    Bennett ML, Fleischer AB, Jr., Chamlin SL, Frieden IJ. Oral corticosteroid use is effective for cutaneous hemangiomas: an evidence-based evaluation. *Arch Dermatol.* Sep 2001;137(9):1208-1213.

[29]    Melo-Gomes JA. Problems related to systemic glucocorticoid therapy in children. *J Rheumatol Suppl.* Apr 1993;37:35-39.

[30]    Leaute-Labreze C, Dumas de la Roque E, Hubiche T, Boralevi F, Thambo JB, Taieb A. Propranolol for severe hemangiomas of infancy. *N Engl J Med.* Jun 12 2008;358(24):2649-2651.

[31]    Price CJ, Lattouf C, Baum B, *et al.* Propranolol *vs.* Corticosteroids for Infantile Hemangiomas: A Multicenter Retrospective Analysis. *Arch Dermatol.* Dec 2011;147(12):1371-1376.

[32]    Artman M, Grayson M, Boerth RC. Propranolol in children: safety-toxicity. *Pediatrics.* Jul 1982;70(1):30-31.

[33]    Sans V, de la Roque ED, Berge J, *et al.* Propranolol for severe infantile hemangiomas: follow-up report. *Pediatrics.* Sep 2009;124(3):e423-431.

[34]    Buckmiller LM, Munson PD, Dyamenahalli U, Dai Y, Richter GT. Propranolol for infantile hemangiomas: early experience at a tertiary vascular anomalies center. *Laryngoscope.* Apr 2010;120(4):676-681.

[35]    Menezes MD, McCarter R, Greene EA, Bauman NM. Status of propranolol for treatment of infantile hemangioma and description of a randomized clinical trial. *Ann Otol Rhinol Laryngol.* Oct 2011;120(10):686-695.

[36]    Drolet BA, Frommelt PC, Chamlin SL, Haggstrom A, Bauman NM, Chiu YE, *et al.* Initiation and use of propranolol for infantile hemangioma: report of a consensus conference. *Pediatrics.* 2013 Jan;131(1):128-40

[37]    Manunza F, Syed S, Laguda B, *et al.* Propranolol for complicated infantile haemangiomas: a case series of 30 infants. *Br J Dermatol.* Feb 1;162(2):466-468.

[38]    Zvulunov A, McCuaig C, Frieden IJ, *et al.* Oral propranolol therapy for infantile hemangiomas beyond the proliferation phase: a multicenter retrospective study. *Pediatr Dermatol.* Mar-Apr;28(2):94-98.

[39]    Blatt J, Morrell DS, Buck S, *et al.* beta-blockers for infantile hemangiomas: a single-institution experience. *Clin Pediatr (Phila).* Aug;50(8):757-763.

[40]    Ni N, Langer P, Wagner R, Guo S. Topical timolol for periocular hemangioma: report of further study. *Arch Ophthalmol.* Mar;129(3):377-379.

[41]    Pope E, Chakkittakandiyil A. Topical timolol gel for infantile hemangiomas: a pilot study. *Arch Dermatol.* May;146(5):564-565.

[42]    Bauman NM, Burke DK, Smith RJ. Treatment of massive or life-threatening hemangiomas with recombinant alpha(2a)-interferon. *Otolaryngol Head Neck Surg.* Jul 1997;117(1):99-110.

[43]    Michaud AP, Bauman NM, Burke DK, Manaligod JM, Smith RJ. Spastic diplegia and other motor disturbances in infants receiving interferon-alpha. *Laryngoscope.* Jul 2004;114(7):1231-1236.

[44]    Le Huu AR, Jokinen CH, Rubin BP, *et al.* Expression of prox1, lymphatic endothelial nuclear transcription factor, in Kaposiform hemangioendothelioma and tufted angioma. *Am J Surg Pathol.* Nov;34(11):1563-1573.

[45]    Alberola FT, Betlloch I, Montero LC, Nortes IB, Martinez NL, Paz AM. Congenital tufted angioma: Case report and review of the literature. *Dermatol Online J.*16(5):2.

[46]    Yesudian PD, Klafkowski J, Parslew R, Gould D, Lloyd D, Pizer B. Tufted angioma-associated Kasabach-Merritt syndrome treated with embolization and vincristine. *Plast Reconstr Surg.* Apr 1 2007;119(4):1392-1393.

[47]    Lyons LL, North PE, Mac-Moune Lai F, Stoler MH, Folpe AL, Weiss SW. Kaposiform hemangioendothelioma: a study of 33 cases emphasizing its pathologic, immunophenotypic, and biologic uniqueness from juvenile hemangioma. *Am J Surg Pathol.* May 2004;28(5):559-568.

[48]    Mukerji SS, Osborn AJ, Roberts J, Valdez TA. Kaposiform hemangioendothelioma (with Kasabach Merritt syndrome) of the head and neck: case report and review of the literature. *Int J Pediatr Otorhinolaryngol.* Oct 2009;73(10):1474-1476.

[49]    Kim T, Roh MR, Cho S, Chung KY. Kasabach-merritt syndrome arising from tufted angioma successfully treated with systemic corticosteroid. *Ann Dermatol.* Nov;22(4):426-430.

[50]    Barabash-Neila R, Garcia-Rodriguez E, Bernabeu-Wittel J, Bueno-Rodriguez I, Ramirez-Villar G, Lopez-Gutierrez JC. Kaposiform Hemangioendothelioma with Kasabach-Merritt phenomenon: Successful Treatment with Vincristine and Ticlopidine. *Indian J Pediatr.* Oct 2012; 79(10):1386-1387.

[51]    Jiang RS, Hu R. Successful treatment of Kasabach-Merritt syndrome arising from kaposiform hemangioendothelioma by systemic corticosteroid therapy and surgery. *Int J Clin Oncol.* Oct 2012;17(5):512-6;17.

[52]    Hermans DJ, van Beynum IM, van der Vijver RJ, Kool LJ, de Blaauw I, van der Vleuten CJ. Kaposiform hemangioendothelioma with Kasabach-Merritt syndrome: a new indication for propranolol treatment. *J Pediatr Hematol Oncol.* May;33(4):e171-173.

[53]    Lopez V, Marti N, Pereda C, *et al.* Successful management of Kaposiform hemangioendothelioma with Kasabach-Merritt phenomenon using vincristine and ticlopidine. *Pediatr Dermatol.* May-Jun 2009;26(3):365-366.

[54]    Hauer J, Graubner U, Konstantopoulos N, Schmidt S, Pfluger T, Schmid I. Effective treatment of kaposiform hemangioendotheliomas associated with Kasabach-Merritt phenomenon using four-drug regimen. *Pediatr Blood Cancer.* Nov 2007;49(6):852-854.

[55]    Hu B, Lachman R, Phillips J, Peng SK, Sieger L. Kasabach-Merritt syndrome-associated kaposiform hemangioendothelioma successfully treated with cyclophosphamide, vincristine, and actinomycin D. *J Pediatr Hematol Oncol.* Nov-Dec 1998;20(6):567-569.

[56]    Blatt J, Stavas J, Moats-Staats B, Woosley J, Morrell DS. Treatment of childhood kaposiform hemangioendothelioma with sirolimus. *Pediatr Blood Cancer.* Dec 15;55(7):1396-1398.

[57]    Smith RJ. Lymphatic malformations. *Lymphat Res Biol.* 2004;2(1):25-31.

[58]    Smith MC, Zimmerman MB, Burke DK, Bauman NM, Sato Y, Smith RJ. Efficacy and safety of OK-432 immunotherapy of lymphatic malformations. *Laryngoscope.* Jan 2009;119(1):107-115.

[59]    Fageeh N, Manoukian J, Tewfik T, Schloss M, Williams HB, Gaskin D. Management of head and neck lymphatic malformations in children. *J Otolaryngol.* Aug 1997;26(4):253-258.

[60]    Emery PJ, Bailey CM, Evans JN. Cystic hygroma of the head and neck. A review of 37 cases. *J Laryngol Otol.* Jun 1984;98(6):613-619.

[61]    de Serres LM, Sie KC, Richardson MA. Lymphatic malformations of the head and neck. A proposal for staging. *Arch Otolaryngol Head Neck Surg.* May 1995;121(5):577-582.

[62]    Giguere CM, Bauman NM, Sato Y, *et al.* Treatment of lymphangiomas with OK-432 (Picibanil) sclerotherapy: a prospective multi-institutional trial. *Arch Otolaryngol Head Neck Surg.* Oct 2002;128(10):1137-1144.

[63]    Smith RJ, Burke DK, Sato Y, Poust RI, Kimura K, Bauman NM. OK-432 therapy for lymphangiomas. *Arch Otolaryngol Head Neck Surg.* Nov 1996;122(11):1195-1199.

[64]    Burrows PE, Mitri RK, Alomari A, *et al.* Percutaneous sclerotherapy of lymphatic malformations with doxycycline. *Lymphat Res Biol.* 2008;6(3-4):209-216.

[65]    Nehra D, Jacobson L, Barnes P, Mallory B, Albanese CT, Sylvester KG. Doxycycline sclerotherapy as primary treatment of head and neck lymphatic malformations in children. *J Pediatr Surg.* Mar 2008;43(3):451-460.

[66]    Impellizzeri P, Romeo C, Borruto FA, *et al.* Sclerotherapy for cervical cystic lymphatic malformations in children. Our experience with computed tomography-guided 98% sterile ethanol insertion and a review of the literature. *J Pediatr Surg.* Dec;45(12):2473-2478.

[67]    Orvidas LJ, Kasperbauer JL. Pediatric lymphangiomas of the head and neck. *Ann Otol Rhinol Laryngol.* Apr 2000;109(4):411-421.

[68]    Happle R. What is a capillary malformation? *J Am Acad Dermatol.* Dec 2008;59(6):1077-1079.

[69]    Shih IH, Lin JY, Chen CH, Hong HS. A birthmark survey in 500 newborns: clinical observation in two northern Taiwan medical center nurseries. *Chang Gung Med J.* May-Jun 2007;30(3):220-225.

[70]    Piram M, Lorette G, Sirinelli D, Herbreteau D, Giraudeau B, Maruani A. Sturge-weber syndrome in patients with facial port-wine stain. *Pediatr Dermatol.* Jan;29(1):32-37.

[71]    Eerola I, Boon LM, Mulliken JB, *et al.* Capillary malformation-arteriovenous malformation, a new clinical and genetic disorder caused by RASA1 mutations. *Am J Hum Genet.* Dec 2003;73(6):1240-1249.

[72]    Oduber CE, van der Horst CM, Hennekam RC. Klippel-Trenaunay syndrome: diagnostic criteria and hypothesis on etiology. *Ann Plast Surg.* Feb 2008;60(2):217-223.

[73]    Berenguer B, Burrows PE, Zurakowski D, Mulliken JB. Sclerotherapy of craniofacial venous malformations: complications and results. *Plast Reconstr Surg.* Jul 1999;104(1):1-11; discussion 12-15.

[74]   Mason KP, Michna E, Zurakowski D, Koka BV, Burrows PE. Serum ethanol levels in children and adults after ethanol embolization or sclerotherapy for vascular anomalies. *Radiology.* Oct 2000;217(1):127-132.

[75]   Kohout MP, Hansen M, Pribaz JJ, Mulliken JB. Arteriovenous malformations of the head and neck: natural history and management. *Plast Reconstr Surg.* Sep 1998;102(3):643-654.

[76]   Liu AS, Mulliken JB, Zurakowski D, Fishman SJ, Greene AK. Extracranial arteriovenous malformations: natural progression and recurrence after treatment. *Plast Reconstr Surg.* Apr;125(4):1185-1194.

# Author Index

# Subject Index

* 9 7 8 1 6 0 8 0 5 1 2 4 3 *